Improving Quality of Care in Family Planning

Jay Satia · Kavita Chauhan

Improving Quality of Care in Family Planning

A Research and Advocacy Agenda for India

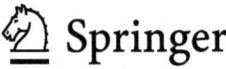

Jay Satia
Indian Institute of Public Health
 Gandhinagar
Gandhinagar, Gujarat
India

Kavita Chauhan
Public Health Foundation of India
Gurgaon
India

ISBN 978-981-10-8131-6   ISBN 978-981-10-8132-3 (eBook)
https://doi.org/10.1007/978-981-10-8132-3

Library of Congress Control Number: 2018930129

© Springer Nature Singapore Pte Ltd. 2018
This work is subject to copyright. All rights are reserved by the Publisher, whether the whole or part of the material is concerned, specifically the rights of translation, reprinting, reuse of illustrations, recitation, broadcasting, reproduction on microfilms or in any other physical way, and transmission or information storage and retrieval, electronic adaptation, computer software, or by similar or dissimilar methodology now known or hereafter developed.
The use of general descriptive names, registered names, trademarks, service marks, etc. in this publication does not imply, even in the absence of a specific statement, that such names are exempt from the relevant protective laws and regulations and therefore free for general use.
The publisher, the authors and the editors are safe to assume that the advice and information in this book are believed to be true and accurate at the date of publication. Neither the publisher nor the authors or the editors give a warranty, express or implied, with respect to the material contained herein or for any errors or omissions that may have been made. The publisher remains neutral with regard to jurisdictional claims in published maps and institutional affiliations.

Printed on acid-free paper

This Springer imprint is published by the registered company Springer Nature Singapore Pte Ltd. part of Springer Nature
The registered company address is: 152 Beach Road, #21-01/04 Gateway East, Singapore 189721, Singapore

Foreword I

Providing high-quality health care services is critical. Quality of care in family planning services is even more important as the users of family planning services differ from other users of health services in one important respect. They are not sick patients. Besides, a large number of them are women and require gender-sensitive services. Also, they are often in the age group of 20–40 years, whereas most patients are older. Finally, young people need youth-friendly services.

Among many priorities in public health, reducing the unmet need for contraception is currently a significant area for the government, multilateral initiatives, non-governmental organizations, and civil society organizations. Unmet need may result in mistimed or unwanted pregnancies which not only adversely affect the mother's and child's health but also stress families.

Recent global research shows that the provision of quality family planning services can reduce unmet need by increasing uptake, prevalence, and continuation of contraception. As access to family planning services is improving and fertility levels are reaching near-replacement levels, improving quality of care in family planning in India has catalysed discourse over the past couple of years. Policy makers recognize that health is essential to economic development and that India's healthy young population provides a demographic window of opportunity for accelerated economic growth. Simultaneously, Indian civil society organizations continue to advocate for quality standards in provision of family planning services and people's right to quality of care.

The Government of India, non-governmental organizations, and the private sector have taken several steps to improve quality standards for providing care to men and women seeking family planning services in India. But as research and experience show, much remains to be done. Research can provide evidence-based guidance on effective and efficient ways to improve quality of care. It is important to expand the knowledge base to take into account people's perspectives, their perceptions of current quality of care, and provider perspectives on provision of services to increase uptake and continuation of contraception and improve the health of couples and their families.

Therefore, the Public Health Foundation of India with support from the David and Lucile Packard Foundation and the Bill and Melinda Gates Foundation has developed this monograph on key research priorities to accelerate progress on improving quality of care in family planning in India. In this process, it not only reviews the research done in India but also draws upon reported experiences of improving quality of care in family planning in India, as well as a Delphi study.

This monograph also includes a report of the consultation on ways to increase demand for quality of care. Most of the current effort on improving quality of care is focused on service provision. However, it is important that users of family planning services are enabled, motivated, and empowered to demand quality of care. Only then can high quality of care be sustained.

I hope this book will be a useful tool for researchers, the government, and non-governmental agencies to chart a path for their efforts towards strengthening quality of care in family planning.

New Delhi, India

K. Srinath Reddy
President
Public Health Foundation of India

Foreword II

The 2012 London Summit on Family Planning reinvigorated the global interest in and commitment to family planning and quality. The Ministry of Health and Family Welfare (MOHFW) of India has issued its own document entitled *India's Vision FP2020*, which outlines strategies to be followed to achieve the stated goal of reaching 48 million additional women with modern contraceptive methods by 2020. A focus on ensuring quality of services is included among these strategies.

Interest in quality, however, is not new. More than 25 years ago, Judith Bruce articulated a client-centred quality of care framework in 1990 to encourage international family planning programmes to move away from a completely demographic rationale of family planning and start paying attention to individual well-being. The 1994 International Conference on Population and Development held in Cairo reaffirmed interest in individual well-being, quality, and reproductive health. The global interest in family planning dwindled for some time for many reasons, including a shift in focus on addressing the HIV epidemic and reducing maternal morbidity and mortality. At present, while the term "quality" is included in the lexicon of family planning, efforts to improve and deliver services of good quality have been mixed.

It is this context that gives me a special pleasure to write the foreword for this book by Jay Satia and Kavita Chauhan of the Public Health Foundation of India. This monograph comes at an important juncture of the family planning programme in India and draws attention to quality of care. It consists of nine chapters which are based on review of research studies and actions taken to improve quality of care in India since 1994. In addition, the authors undertook two rounds of Delphi study to identify high-priority research, action, and advocacy needs. The last chapter is based on a consultation held in Jodhpur which focused on creating demand for quality of care in India.

Improving quality of services in a complex system like India is quite challenging. Many of the steps and interventions required to improve quality are recognized and discussed in this monograph. While implementing these policy- and programme-level interventions, it will be important to focus continuously on the quality of care received by the clients whenever they come into contact with any service provider offering family planning information and service—either at a health facility or during service outreach. It is how clients are treated and what care they receive which is important in influencing their subsequent contraceptive and fertility behaviour.

We can always think of educating clients and communities to demand services of good quality. However, from the programmatic perspective, what is done to improve the motivation and behaviour of service providers will determine their behaviour towards clients of services. Many interventions, e.g., method-specific targets for providers and sterilization camps, implemented in the past had adversely affected the quality of care received by the clients. While these interventions have now been discontinued, a system of monetary incentives for providers and clients remains in place. It is important to assess the implication of this system for quality of care received by clients. An important component of improving quality of care is to periodically monitor quality of care received by clients, especially whenever changes in the programme are made that would influence the behaviour of providers.

Information received by clients at the time of initiating contraception is an important component of quality of care. Data analysed from the National Family Health Survey (NFHS-3) showed that only 16% of current contraceptive users reported receiving information at the time they initiated contraception (during five years prior to the interview) on all three elements—other contraceptive options, side effects of the method selected, and how to manage these side effects if they occur. Moreover, only two out of three sterilized women reported that they were told that sterilization is permanent. Admittedly, these indicators do not reflect the entire content of client–provider interactions and must have improved by now, but they are unlikely to have reached a level of 80 or 100%.

It is essential to accelerate progress on improving the quality of care received by family planning clients in India because clients have a right to receive good quality, and good quality also contributes to the achievement of other desirable reproductive health outcomes. In order to improve the quality of care, it is important to identify interventions to improve quality and to develop a research and advocacy agenda relevant to the Indian context. This monograph makes important contributions in all three areas. It has identified eight important areas of research, including a focus on clients, providers, and measurement of quality of care.

I trust that the monograph will be of interest not only to researchers and academic institutions, but also to programme managers, policy makers, and advocacy organizations. A concerted effort by all concerned in improving the quality of care in the family planning programme in India will contribute to the achievement of FP2020 goals and will help the MOHFW to complete the transition, mentioned in India's FP2020 document, from a "population control centric approach" to a "reproductive rights based approach". Above all, such an approach will enhance individual well-being and empower individuals to achieve their reproductive intentions safely.

New York, US

Anrudh K. Jain, Ph.D.
Distinguished Scholar
Population Council

Acknowledgements

This book is an effort to take forward the ongoing discourse on the important issue of quality of care in family planning, and to identify the research and advocacy priorities for India. We believe that providing quality care to women and couples seeking family planning and contraception services (particularly for birth spacing) will enable scale-up of interventions to strengthen reach and coverage of the family planning programme.

The David and Lucile Packard Foundation and the Bill and Melinda Gates Foundation provided generous support for this project, without which this book would not have been possible. We are grateful to Anand Sinha, Tamara Karenin, and Lana Dakan from the David and Lucile Packard Foundation and Sandhya Venkateswaran, Lester Coutinho, and Richa Shankar from the Bill and Melinda Gates Foundation for their guidance and encouragement.

To provide strategic guidance to this effort, a Steering Group on Quality of Care in Family Planning was set up with representation from key stakeholders. This group was chaired by Rakesh Kumar, former Joint Secretary, Reproductive and Child Health, Ministry of Health and Family Welfare (MoHFW), Government of India, with S. K. Sikdar, Deputy Commissioner, Family Planning, MoHFW as its convener. We express our gratitude to them for their support. The purpose of this group was to review evidence on "what works", to identify issues that need further research, and to strengthen discourse around quality of care in family planning.

The book is based on our review of existing knowledge on this topic (research and experiences which represent the work of individuals, different partner organizations, and the national and state governments), a Delphi exercise, and discussions with stakeholders working on family planning in India. We greatly appreciate the support of key individuals, who are mentioned below, in helping us with background information and sharing their perspectives with us:

Aarushi Khanna, Aditi Iyer, Ahana Sood, Alok Banerjee, Alok Vajpayee, Amit Bhanot, Amit Shan, Anchita Patil, Anjali Sen, Anupam Shukla, Aparajita Gogoi, Arnab Dey, Bhartendu Sharma, Deepa Nag Chowdhury, Devika Biswas, Dinesh Aggarwal, Elizabeth Salazar, Fauzdar Ram, Geeta Sethi, Gita Pillai, Ipsita Parida,

Jameel Zamir, Jayanta K. Das, Joanna Percher, Jyoti Vajpayee, Kalpana Apte, Karen Hardee, Kirti Iyengar, M. E. Khan, Madhubala Nath, Manak Matiyani, Manju Katoch, Mansiha Bhise, Nayla Shakeel, Niranjan Saggurti, Nirmala Murthy, Paromita Vohra, Poonam Mutterja, Pragati Singh, Pranita Achyut, Preeti Anand, Pritpal Marjara, Priya Nanda, Rashmi Kukreja, Ravi Anand, Ravi Verma, Rupsa Malik, Sachin Kothari, Sandhya Gautam, Sanghita Bhattacharya, Shanti Mahendra, Sharad Agarwal, Shilpa John, Shriram Haridass, Shubhra Phillips, Sonalini Mirchandani, Sudha Tewari, Sulbha Swaroop, Suneeta Mittal, Teja Ram, Vinoj Manning, V. K. Mathur, V. S. Chandrasekhar, and Yeme Belayneh.

We are grateful to the unknown reviewers whose prescriptive comments helped us refine some of the sections of the book.

We thank K. Srinath Reddy, President, PHFI, for supporting us in this effort and for writing a foreword, and Anrudh K. Jain for his valuable inputs and for writing a second foreword to introduce this important topic.

Finally, we are grateful to Springer for being the publisher of this book. We thank Shinjini Chatterjee, Priya Vyas and the editorial team for assisting us through their able support.

Gujarat, India	Jay Satia
Gurgaon, India	Kavita Chauhan
August 2017	

Contents

1 **The Need to Improve Quality of Care in India's Family Planning** 1
   1.1   Introduction 1
   1.2   Quality of Care is Critical in Family Planning 3
   1.3   Need to Accelerate Improvements in Quality of Care in Family Planning 4
   1.4   Description of the Project 6
   1.5   Approach for Developing Background Paper 7
   References 10

2 **What is Quality? Quality of Care Frameworks** 13
   2.1   Donabedian's Quality of Care Framework 13
   2.2   Quality Improvement in the Health Sector 15
         2.2.1   Measurement of Quality 15
         2.2.2   Quality Improvement 16
   2.3   Reproductive, Maternal, Newborn, Child, and Adolescent Health: Strategy and Quality of Care 16
   2.4   National Quality Assurance Programme 17
   2.5   Quality of Care Frameworks for Family Planning 19
   2.6   Rights of Clients and Providers 20
   2.7   Quality of Care as a Right of Clients 21
   2.8   Incorporating Health System and Community Influences in Quality of Care Framework 25
   2.9   A Proposed Comprehensive Framework for Interventions to Improve Quality of Care 27
   References 29

3 Steps Taken by the Government of India to Improve Quality of Care 33
3.1 Guidelines Developed by the Government of India to Ensure Quality in Family Planning Service Delivery 33
3.2 Family Planning Indemnity Scheme 36
3.3 Quality Assurance Committees 36
3.4 Expanding Contraceptive Choice and Improving Access 37
3.5 Improving Quality of Care in Government Service Delivery with Support from NGOs and Development Partners 37
3.5.1 Strengthening Systems 37
3.5.2 Public–Private Collaboration for Comprehensive Improvement of Quality of Care in Government Services 39
3.5.3 Improving Provider Competence for Intrauterine Contraceptive Devices and Non-scalpel Vasectomy 43
3.6 Other Efforts to Improve Quality of Care 45
3.6.1 EngenderHealth: Improving Quality at Service Sites Through Quality Circles (COPE) 45
3.6.2 Creating Demand for Family Planning to Improve Quality of Care: The Innovations in Family Planning Services Project 46
3.7 Integration of Family Planning Services with Other Health Services 47
3.8 Current Status of Implementation of Quality of Care Improvement Efforts: Perspectives from the Field 47
3.8.1 Visit to Department of Health and Family Welfare, Government of Rajasthan (May 2016) 47
3.8.2 Visit to Department of Health and Family Welfare, Government of Uttar Pradesh (April 2016) 49
3.9 Conclusion 51
References 52

4 Steps Taken by NGOs and the Private Sector to Improve Quality of Care 53
4.1 Quality Improvement Interventions in NGO-Led Innovations 53
4.1.1 Respond: Project on Scaling up of Non-scalpel Vasectomy 53
4.1.2 FHI 360: PROGRESS (Programme Research for Strengthening Services) 54
4.1.3 Ujjwal Project 54
4.1.4 Population Council: Systematic Screening to Integrate Reproductive Health Services in India 55
4.1.5 The Dimpa Programme 56

		4.1.6	Improving Quality of Care of Service Delivery for Intrauterine Contraceptive Devices	57
		4.1.7	Odisha Urban Reproductive Health Project	57
	4.2	Other Projects in the NGO Sector		58
		4.2.1	Parivar Seva Sansthan	58
		4.2.2	Marie Stopes India	58
		4.2.3	Action Research and Training for Health	59
		4.2.4	Population Services International	60
		4.2.5	Public Health Foundation of India, United Nations Population Fund, and Federation of Obstetric and Gynaecological Societies of India	61
		4.2.6	Addressing the Needs of Young People: Empowerment Through Life Skills Education and Counselling	61
		4.2.7	mHealth for Content Distribution	62
		4.2.8	Empowering Clients to Demand Quality of Care for Maternal Health Using Mobile Technology: A Pilot Study in Jharkhand	63
		4.2.9	Pehel: Addressing Women's Health in Rajasthan, Delhi, and Uttar Pradesh	63
		4.2.10	Family Planning Association of India SETU Core+ Project	65
		4.2.11	DKT India	66
	4.3	Approaches to Assuring Quality of Care in Social Franchising Operations		66
		4.3.1	Social Franchising Programmes in India	67
		4.3.2	Ensuring Quality of Care in Social Franchising Operations	67
		4.3.3	Devising a Quality Metric for Social Franchisee Operations in Family Planning Globally	68
	4.4	Social Marketing		69
	4.5	Advocating Reproductive Choices: Catalysing Stakeholder Engagement for Repositioning Family Planning		70
	4.6	Conclusion and the Way Forward		70
	References			72
5	**Review of Research Studies**			75
	5.1	Introduction		75
	5.2	Review of Quality of Care Around 1994		76
		5.2.1	Clients' Perspectives	76
		5.2.2	Provider Perspectives	76
		5.2.3	Improving Quality of Care	77
	5.3	Studies Since 1995 on the Quality of Care Provided		77

	5.4	Status of Quality of Care	78
	5.5	Informed Choice and Discontinuation Rates	81
	5.6	Service Quality for Adolescent and Young People	83
	5.7	Intervention to Improve Quality of Care	83
		5.7.1 Facility-Level Interventions	84
		5.7.2 Programme-Level Interventions	85
		5.7.3 Community-Level Interventions	85
	5.8	Factors Influencing Quality of Care	87
	5.9	Impact of Improved Quality of Care	89
	5.10	Research Methodologies Used	90
	5.11	Global Reviews on Quality of Care in Family Planning	91
	5.12	Recent Relevant International Research on Quality of Care	93
	References	99
6	**Consensus Building on Quality of Care Priorities**	105
	6.1	Methodology of Delphi Process	105
	6.2	Research Agenda: Summary of Findings from First Round Delphi	107
		6.2.1 Research Agenda: Questions Rated as High Priority by Respondents and Key Inputs Received	108
		6.2.2 Research Agenda: Questions Rated as Medium Priority by Respondents and Key Inputs Received	109
		6.2.3 Research Agenda: Questions Rated as Low Priority by Respondents and Key Inputs Received	111
	6.3	Action Agenda	113
		6.3.1 Questions Rated as High Priority by Respondents and Key Inputs Received	113
		6.3.2 Questions Rated as Low Priority by Respondents and Key Inputs Received	114
	6.4	Advocacy Agenda: Key Findings of Delphi First Round	115
		6.4.1 Most Recommended Priorities and Key Inputs Received from Respondents	116
		6.4.2 Questions Rated as Low Priority and Key Inputs Received from Respondents	116
	6.5	Research Agenda: Summary of Findings from Second Round of Delphi	116
	6.6	Conclusion	118
	Reference	118
7	**Operationalizing the Action and Advocacy Agenda for Quality of Care**	119
	7.1	Introduction	119
	7.2	The Need to Augment Action on the Ground	120
	7.3	Operationalizing the Action Agenda	121

		7.3.1	Activating Quality of Care Organizational Mechanisms.................................	121
		7.3.2	Enhancing the Accountability of the Programme	123
		7.3.3	Improving Supplies	124
	7.4	Other Actions Identified as Relatively Lower Priority	126
		7.4.1	Improving Training	126
		7.4.2	Strengthening the Role of ASHAs.................	126
		7.4.3	Quality of Care in the Private Sector...............	126
		7.4.4	Periodic Assessment of Quality of Care............	127
	7.5	Accelerating Advocacy for Improving Quality of Care	127
	7.6	Past and Present Advocacy Efforts.......................	128
		7.6.1	NGO-Led Advocacy Efforts Promoting Repositioning of Family Planning in India	128
		7.6.2	*Legal Instruments*: Devika Biswas v. Union of India & Ors (WP [C] 95/2012)	129
		7.6.3	Social Audit as an Instrument to Improve Family Planning Services in Uttar Pradesh, 2001–2005	129
	7.7	What Is Needed to Advance the Advocacy Agenda for Quality of Care in Family Planning in India?....................	130
	7.8	Key Focus Areas for Advocacy..........................	131
	References			132

8 **Developing a Research Agenda for Accelerating Progress on Improving Quality of Care** 133
	8.1	Need to Accelerate Improvements in Quality of Care	133
	8.2	What Has Been Done to Improve Quality of Care?	134
	8.3	Review of Research Studies	134
	8.4	Findings of the Delphi Study..........................	135
	8.5	Emerging Research Agenda...........................	136
	8.6	Operationalizing the Research Agenda...................	137
		8.6.1	Client Perceptions of the Quality of Care Being Provided	137
		8.6.2	Improving Quality of Care in Adolescent/Youth Family Planning Services	140
		8.6.3	Enabling and Motivating Providers to Provide Quality of Care	141
		8.6.4	Effect of Health System Operations Influencing Quality of Care in Family Planning.....................	143
		8.6.5	Political, Legal, and Organizational Context of the Health System	144
		8.6.6	Activating Organizational Mechanisms to Improve Quality of Care	144
		8.6.7	Quality of Care Metrics, Monitoring System, and Enhancing Accountability....................	145

		8.6.8	Ensuring Quality of Care While Introducing Additional Methods	149
		8.6.9	Benefits of Improved Quality of Care	150
	8.7	Summary and Conclusion		152
	References			154
9	**Enhancing Demand for Quality of Care in Family Planning in India: A Consultation Report**			157
	9.1	Why Focus on Enhancing Demand for Quality of Care?		157
	9.2	What Does the Available Evidence Indicate?		158
	9.3	Clients at the Centre of Quality of Care		160
		9.3.1	Client Perspectives	160
		9.3.2	Empowering Clients	161
	9.4	Empowering Young People to Demand Quality of Care		161
		9.4.1	Service-Seeking Behaviour of Young People	161
		9.4.2	Unpacking Youth-Friendly Health Services	162
	9.5	Engaging Community		162
		9.5.1	Influencing Societal Norms	162
		9.5.2	Mainstreaming Community Involvement	163
	9.6	Working with Other Sectors		164
	9.7	Communication for Enhancing Demand		164
	9.8	Governance		165
	9.9	Accountability		166
		9.9.1	Accountability for What and Why	166
		9.9.2	Whose Accountability and to Whom	166
		9.9.3	Institutionalizing Accountability	168
	9.10	Advocacy		168
		9.10.1	Evidence Base for Advocacy	169
		9.10.2	Process of Advocacy	170
	9.11	Service Provision		170
		9.11.1	Health System	170
		9.11.2	Empowering Providers	172
	9.12	Conclusion		172
	References			173

Annexure 1: Delphi Questionnaire 175

Annexure 2: Clients at the Centre of Quality of Care 181

Annexure 3: Community Engagement for Demanding Quality of Care in Family Planning 183

Annexure 4: Interventions/Research for Creating Demand for Quality of Care by Clients 187

Annexure 5: Enhancing Programme Accountability for Quality of Care 189

Annexure 6: Evidence-Based Advocacy to Support Demand for Quality of Care 193

About the Authors

Jay Satia is a former Professor of the Indian Institute of Management Ahmedabad (IIMA) where he taught for more than 20 years, and served as its Dean during 1987–1989. At IIMA, he worked on operations management as well as on management of health, population, and nutrition programmes. During the period 1993–2008, he was the Executive Director of the International Council on Management of Population Programmes, a Malaysia-based international non-governmental organization dedicated to seeking excellence in management of population programmes through leadership and management development. At present, he is Emeritus Professor at the Indian Institute of Public Health Gandhinagar. He has several publications to his credit on management, leadership, and population issues and has held a range of management and board of directors positions in various Indian and international organizations. He holds a B.E. from Bombay University and an MS and Ph.D. in industrial engineering from Stanford University, USA.

Kavita Chauhan is a behavioural science professional at the Public Health Foundation of India. She has over 14 years of experience in designing and managing strategic health communication and advocacy initiatives, research on behaviour change, and capacity building on public health communications. Her previous work at CARE India integrated planning and implementing strategies related to reproductive health needs of communities with a special focus on young people. At Futures Group Inc., under the global POLICY Project, she formulated HIV/AIDS policy interventions with the government, faith-based organizations, and NGOs, and facilitated decentralized planning for HIV/AIDS and maternal health efforts. She holds a BA in English literature and MA in social work from Jamia Millia Islamia, New Delhi, and an M.Sc. in public health from the London School of Hygiene and Tropical Medicine (LSHTM). Currently she is enrolled as a research degree student at LSHTM.

Abbreviations

ANM	Auxiliary nurse midwife
ARTH	Action Research and Training for Health
ASHA	Accredited social health activist
BCC	Behaviour change communication
CAC	Comprehensive abortion care
CBD	Community-based distributor
CHARM	Counselling Husbands to Achieve RH and Marital Equity
CHC	Community health centre
COPE	Client-oriented, provider-efficient
CSO	Civil society organization
DLHS	District Level Household Survey
DMPA	Depo-Provera or depot medroxyprogesterone acetate
DQAC	District quality assurance committee
DQAG	District quality assurance group
ECP	Emergency contraceptive pills
ELA	Expected level of achievement
FOGSI	Federation of Obstetrics and Gynaecology Societies of India
FP	Family planning
HLFPPT	Hindustan Latex Family Planning Promotion Trust
HMIS	Hospital management information system
HTSP	Healthy Timing and Spacing of Pregnancy
ICPD	International Conference on Population and Development
ICRW	International Center for Research on Women
IEC	Information education communication
IFPS	Innovations in Family Planning Services
IPHS	Indian Public Health Standards
IPPF	International Planned Parenthood Federation
IUCD	Intrauterine contraceptive device
IUD	Intrauterine device

IVRS	Interactive Voice Response System
JHPIEGO	Johns Hopkins Program for International Education in Gynecology and Obstetrics
LAM	Lactational amenorrhea method
LARC	Long-acting reversible contraception
mCPR	Contraception prevalence rate by modern methods
MNCH	Maternal, neonatal, and child health
MoHFW	Ministry of Health and Family Welfare
MSI	Marie Stopes India
NFHS	National Family Health Survey
NGO	Non-governmental Organization
NHM	National Health Mission
NHSRC	National Health Systems Resource Centre
NQAP	National Quality Assurance Programme
NRHM	National Rural Health Mission
NSV	Non-scalpel vasectomy
OCP	Oral contraceptive pills
PFI	Population Foundation of India
PHC	Primary health centre
PHFI	Public Health Foundation of India
PIP	Programme implementation plan
POP	Progesterone-only pills
PPFP	Postpartum family planning
PPIUCD	Postpartum intrauterine contraceptive device
PPP	Public–private partnership
PSI	Population Services International
PSS	Parivar Seva Sansthan
QA	Quality assurance
QAC	Quality assurance committee
QI	Quality improvement
QoC	Quality of care
RH	Reproductive health
RHCLMIS	Reproductive health commodities logistics management information system
RKS	Rogi Kalyan Samiti
RKSK	Rashtriya Kishor Swasthtya Karyakram
RMNCH+A	Reproductive, maternal, neonatal, child+adolescent health
SDM	Standard Days Method
SQAC	State quality assurance committee
SRH	Sexual and reproductive health
TFR	Total fertility rate
UHI	Urban Health Initiative
UNFPA	United Nations Population Fund

USAID	United States Agency for International Development
VHSNC	Village Health, Sanitation, and Nutrition Committee
WHO	World Health Organization
YFHS	Youth-Friendly Health Services (programme)

List of Figures

Fig. 1.1	A schematic of the background paper	8
Fig. 2.1	Donabedian's quality of care framework	14
Fig. 2.2	Interventions to improve quality	16
Fig. 2.3	Bruce-Jain framework related to Donabedian's framework	20
Fig. 2.4	IPPF's framework on quality of care	22
Fig. 2.5	Framework for voluntary family planning programmes that respect, protect, and fulfil human rights	24
Fig. 2.6	Quality of care to rights-based approach	25
Fig. 2.7	Improving quality of care: systems framework	28
Fig. 6.1	Delphi process	106
Fig. 8.1	Developing a research agenda for accelerating improvements in quality of care	136

List of Tables

Table 2.1	Variables to be influenced to improve quality of care	29
Table 5.1	Research methods used.	91
Table 5.2	A comparison of findings from our review of research studies in india and the global review	92
Table 6.1	Research agenda.	107
Table 6.2	Summary of findings from first round Delphi.	113
Table 6.3	Key findings of the Delphi first round	115
Table 8.1	Potential research areas.	137
Table 8.2	Summary of types of research and potential utility of each research area.	153
Table 9.1	Interventions for enhancing demand for quality of care in family planning	159

Chapter 1
The Need to Improve Quality of Care in India's Family Planning

Abstract This chapter introduces the importance of quality of care in reducing the unmet need for family planning, and the need to accelerate progress on improving quality of care in Indian family planning services. We present a brief overview of the current context, i.e., the FP2020 (global and national) initiative, to highlight the importance of addressing the issue of quality of care. The FP2020 initiative argues for voluntary, rights-based family planning programmes. The rights-based approach to family planning builds on the bedrock of quality of care, which means listening to what women want, treating individuals with dignity and respect, and ensuring that everyone has access to full information and high-quality care.

Keywords FP2020 · Quality of care · Rights-based approach

1.1 Introduction

Interest in family planning (FP) has grown globally in recent years due to the Family Planning 2020 (FP2020) Initiative. It is a global partnership, an outcome of the London Summit on Family Planning held in 2012, that supports the rights of women and girls to decide, freely and for themselves, whether, when, and how many children they want to have. At the 2012 London Summit, 69 countries pledged to bring modern contraception within reach of an additional 120 million women and girls by the year 2020. Achieving the FP2020 goal is seen as a critical milestone to ensuring universal access to sexual and reproductive health (SRH) services and rights by 2030, as laid out in the UN's Sustainable Development Goals 3 (ensure healthy lives and promote well-being for all at all ages) and 5 (achieving gender equality and the empowerment of women and girls).

India has focused on realizing the FP 2020 India-adapted goal of providing FP services to 48 million additional users during the period 2012–2020. This is a large increase compared to an estimated coverage of 100 million users as of 2012, and requires significant reduction in unmet need for FP (MoHFW 2014).

Achieving the goal of 48 million additional users would mean reaching a contraception prevalence rate by modern methods (mCPR) of 63.7%, which would necessitate contributions from all states of India. The government, at national and state levels, has drawn out comprehensive roadmaps and also district action plans adopting a decentralized planning approach focusing on operationalization of facilities and delivery of FP services.

The projections show that the share of the much-preferred female sterilization will decrease substantially and that of spacing methods will increase significantly. The current focus on postpartum family planning (PPFP), and the introduction of a new method in postpartum intrauterine contraceptive devices (PPIUCD) as well as a new intrauterine contraceptive device (IUCD) (Cu 375), will assist in accelerating India's progress towards achieving the FP2020 goals.

The government is taking several initiatives to improve uptake of services and delivery of care. Key FP interventions include the fixed-day strategy, encouraging male participation, and community-based schemes delivered through accredited social health activists (ASHA), viz., home delivery of contraceptives, ensuring spacing at birth, pregnancy testing kits, FP counsellors, compensation scheme, the Family Planning Indemnity Scheme, and public–private partnership initiatives, just to name a few. The government is also harnessing the expertise of various partners in the fields of advocacy, capacity building, communication (information education communication [IEC] and behaviour change communication [BCC]), programme management, quality improvement (QI), evaluation and assessments, feasibility studies, development of resource material and e-learning modules, software development, social marketing, social franchising, and provision of skilled human resources for successful implementation of the programme.

Recently, the Ministry of Health and Family Welfare (MoHFW) has taken several steps to expand the basket of choices. Three new methods have been introduced in the National Family Planning Programme, which include: (*a*) injectable contraceptive Depo-Provera, or depot medroxyprogesterone acetate (DMPA) (Antara)—a three-monthly injection; (*b*) Centchroman pills (Chhaya)—a non-hormonal once-a-week pill; and (*c*) progesterone-only pills (POP) for lactating mothers. In addition, packaging for condoms, oral contraceptive pills (OCP), and emergency contraceptive pills (ECP) has been redesigned and improved so as to increase the demand for these commodities. A new 360-degree, holistic FP campaign with a new logo was launched in 2016 with film actor Amitabh Bachchan as the brand ambassador (MoHFW 2016).

Achieving the above goals would also require working to reduce teenage marriages and teenage births, increasing the literacy of the girl child, and addressing other socio-cultural barriers and underlying determinants that lead to inequities in access to and use of FP. The National Rural Health Mission (NRHM), now the National Health Mission (NHM), also emphasized reproductive, maternal, newborn, child, and adolescent health (RMNCH+A). The RMNCH+A strategy has provided a platform for addressing reproductive rights while integrating the current FP services with maternal, child, as well as adolescent health (FP2020 2014).

1.1 Introduction

Reducing the unmet need is required to realize FP2020 goals as well as to improve the health of women and children in India. First, fewer births would put fewer mothers and infants at risk of mortality. Second, it would lead to fewer unintended pregnancies and unsafe abortions which increase the mortality risk. The FP2020 initiative is expected to avert 23.9 million births, 1 million infant deaths, and over 42,000 maternal deaths by 2020 in India.

Globally, the effect of provision of contraceptive services as part of a reproductive health (RH) package, meeting 90% of the unmet need for contraception, would reduce births by almost 28 million, and consequently avert deaths that could have occurred at 2015 rates of fertility and mortality. Thus, 67,000 maternal deaths, 440,000 neonatal deaths, 473,000 child deaths, and 564,000 stillbirths could be averted from avoided pregnancies worldwide. In comparison, scaling up all
interventions in an integrated package of maternal, newborn, and child health (along with folic acid supplementation, a key RH intervention) in 2015 for the (hypothetical) immediate achievement of 90% coverage would avert 149,000 maternal deaths, 1,498,000 neonatal deaths, 1,515,000 additional child deaths, and 849,000 stillbirths (Black et al. 2016). Thus, reducing unmet need for contraception would result in a third to half of the impact of scaling up maternal, newborn, and child health services (Jain 1989).

1.2 Quality of Care is Critical in Family Planning

The FP2020 initiative argues for voluntary, rights-based FP programmes. A rights-based approach to FP builds on the bedrock of quality of care (QoC), which means listening to what women want, treating individuals with dignity and respect, and ensuring that everyone has access to full information and high-quality care.

Globally, demographic and health surveys in 52 countries between 2005 and 2014 reveal the most common reasons that married women cite for not using contraception despite wanting to avoid a pregnancy (Sedgh et al. 2016). Twenty-six per cent of these women cite concerns about contraceptive side effects and health risks; 24% say that they have sex infrequently or not at all; 23% say that they or others close to them oppose contraception; and 20% report that they are breastfeeding and/or haven't resumed menstruation after giving birth. Women with unmet need for contraception rarely say that they are unaware of contraception, that they do not have access to a source of supply, or that it costs too much. Compared with earlier studies on women's reasons for not using contraception, a larger proportion of women now cite side effects and infrequent sex as reasons for non-use. Contraceptive services should place priority on improving the information and counselling they provide and the range of methods they offer. All sexually active women, whether married or not, need information about their risk of becoming pregnant and about the choices of methods that could meet their needs.

The third round of the National Family Health Survey (NFHS-3 2005–2006) found that excluding fertility-related reasons, method-related reasons accounted for nearly half (47%) of the reasons for non-use of contraception.

There are two categories of women with an unmet need for FP: those who have never used contraception, and those who have used but discontinued it although they continue to have an unmet need. Studies show that improved QoC received at the time of contraceptive initiation has subsequently increased method continuation and reduced unwanted child bearing (Jain et al. 2013). One way to reduce discontinuation is to expand contraceptive choice by increasing availability of and access to multiple methods. A second approach is to improve QoC and client–provider interactions. Several studies show the importance of improved QoC in ensuring continuation. However, the failure to find a significant effect of interventions in randomized control trials has sometimes generated scepticism regarding the role of improved quality in increasing contraceptive continuation. It could be that the QoC at the baseline was already high in these trials, or that the improvement in QoC by the interventions was too small. Nevertheless, a World Health Organization (WHO) study (Ali et al. 2012) stresses the need to improve service quality, particularly counselling, as a means of reducing high discontinuation rate. Jain et al. (2013) recommend that enabling past users with unmet need to resume use, and encouraging current users to continue use of the same or another method, could be an effective strategy to reduce future unmet need.

In view of the predominance of female sterilization in the method mix in India, accounting for 34% of contraceptive use out of a total of 47.1% (MoHFW 2007–2008), discontinuation rates have not received much attention. The District Level Household Survey (2007–2008) (DLHS-3) shows that ever users of any modern method were 55.6% compared to current users at 48% (MoHFW 2012–2013). However, the use of the spacing method is gradually increasing, and FP2020 strategies also seek to increase their use.

Improving QoC will enable women and men to practise contraception safely and effectively. By providing informed choice of contraceptive methods, it will reduce unmet need for FP. By ensuring continuity of care and the appropriate constellation of RH services, it will reduce discontinuation of contraceptive use.

Thus, improving QoC of FP services is critical from the point of view of individual, national and global considerations.

1.3 Need to Accelerate Improvements in Quality of Care in Family Planning

During the last decade, the MoHFW has introduced several measures to improve the quality of FP services. It has issued guidelines for QoC, improved health facilities, increased emphasis on spacing methods by involving ASHAs, expanded choice by promoting non-scalpel vasectomy (NSV) and PPIUCD, appointed counsellors at high-volume health facilities, and increased the focus on adolescents.

The MoHFW has developed guidelines and standards for service delivery. Mandated by the Supreme Court of India in 2005, the government had established quality assurance (QA) structures comprising QA cells and QA committees for ensuring quality in sterilization services (male and female) at state and district levels. The ambit of these committees and cells was subsequently expanded to cover all RMNCH+A services. Technical guidelines for various contraceptive services have also been updated. More recently, the government has asked the National Health Systems Resource Centre (NHSRC) to initiate a process of accreditation of facilities for RMNCH+A services and various disease control programmes. The NHSRC has developed assessment tools and has begun the process for district hospitals, to be extended later to sub-district health facilities. More recently, the government has decided to introduce DMPA, POP, and Saheli (a weekly pill) to expand the choice of contraceptive methods. It has also updated manuals and guidelines.

Progress in improving QoC in FP has been slow, however. Quality of care in FP has been a cause of concern for almost as long as the programme has been operational, and was marked in earlier times by a major emphasis on targets and related incentives. It continues to suffer from lack of or inadequate choice of contraceptive methods resulting in a skewed method mix, weak QA in technical service delivery, and poor interpersonal care. There is some literature on assessing QoC, identifying barriers to improving quality, pilot programmes to improve QoC, and advocacy efforts. Despite investments in infrastructure, human resources, and development of guidelines and protocols, surveys and studies of quality of FP services in Indian programmes have repeatedly shown shortfalls. Therefore, much needs to be done to improve the QoC of FP services.

The Expert Meeting on Improving Quality of FP and Reproductive Health Programme in India, supported by the David and Lucile Packard Foundation, held in Goa in October 2013, argued for evidence-based effective advocacy for QoC in FP. It suggested priority actions for research on the current status of QoC, effective models that impact QoC, identification of best practices and challenges, ways to ensure technical QoC, and an assessment of the impact of incentives and targets on QoC. It also sought innovations in the areas of QoC indicators for FP, strengthening counselling including use of mHealth, models to reach marginalized populations, and ways to involve village health, nutrition, and sanitation committees (VHNSCs) to improve QoC and for government to operationalize QA officer posts and committees at state and district levels. It also emphasized monitoring of QoC including accreditation of health facilities and commodity security.

A recent study, "Quality of Care in Provision of Female Sterilization and IUD Services" (Achyut et al. 2014), supported by the David and Lucile Packard Foundation in Bihar and conducted by the International Center for Research on Women (ICRW), identified several issues pertaining to QoC in FP. A field visit following sterilization deaths in Bilaspur, Chhattisgarh, organized by the Population Foundation of India (PFI 2014), also made several recommendations. Taken together they identified the following:

- *Service delivery*: Improve privacy in facilities; increase number of beds, equipment, drugs and supplies; fill the posts and appoint adequate number of counsellors.
- *Programme practices*: Strengthen counselling and method-specific skills of providers through high-quality clinical training; activate QA officers and QA committees for adherence to and supervision of quality standards; improve monitoring of QoC; manage supply chain for spacing methods; increase resource allocation for improving QoC; include spacing methods; stop system for allotment of expected level of achievement (ELA) and instead ensure access to and counselling for FP services to all couples; and engage communities and women to ensure informed choice.
- *Policy decisions*: Discontinue incentives for providers and motivators and instead use freed-up resources to improve QoC; emphasize monitoring of QoC to achieve balance between focus on quantity and quality; expand basket of choice by introducing additional contraceptive methods in the public sector based upon global and neighbouring-country experiences; carry out comprehensive third-party evaluation of QoC and revise state population policies.

Available data from NFHS-4 (2014–2015) shows, however, that the unmet need for contraception in India declined from 13.9% in NFHS-3 (2005–2006) to 12.9%. Thus, there has been only a marginal decline in unmet need in major states between NFHS-3 (2005–2006) and NFHS-4 (2014–2015). The percentage of users ever told about the side effects of the current method increased from 34.4% in NFHS 3 (2005–2006) to 46.5% in NFHS 4 (2014–2015); only about a 12% point increase in a decade.

Thus, a nearly static unmet need and persistent shortfalls in QoC despite some improvements and recommendation by groups of researchers argue for the need to accelerate improvements in QoC building upon efforts already made or under way.

1.4 Description of the Project

The Public Health Foundation of India (PHFI) received a grant from the David and Lucile Packard Foundation and the Bill and Melinda Gates Foundation to develop a research, action, and advocacy agenda to improve QoC in FP. More specifically, the project was to undertake a background review to synthesize available knowledge and evidence on this issue, and convene a national-level meeting to discuss the issue on a larger platform and propose action and research inputs for taking this work forward.

With a goal of accelerating improvements in QoC of FP services in India, the expected project outcomes are:

1. Research agenda: identify issues that need further research and develop a research agenda.

2. Action agenda: develop and understanding of "what works"—best practices and innovations to address QoC issues.
3. Develop advocacy processes for advancing the QoC discourse in the country.

The above outcomes would be realized by the following activities:

- Preparing a background paper synthesizing knowledge from diverse strands of literature (assessment studies, pilot interventions, evaluations of government actions) to build a research, action, and advocacy agenda;
- A national consultation to discuss QoC issues and propose measures to accelerate progress towards improving QoC in FP in India; and
- Widely disseminating the background paper.

1.5 Approach for Developing Background Paper

We began with the idea that we would synthesize peer-reviewed published research studies in India, identify gaps, and develop a research agenda to bridge this gap. As the International Conference on Population and Development (ICPD) in 1994 was a turning point for the programme, we began our review from 1995. However, we could find very few studies in QoC in FP during the last two decades, from 1995 to 2015. Therefore, we used a diversified approach to prepare this background paper. In addition to a review of research studies, we also reviewed actions taken to improve QoC, as well as carrying out two rounds of Delphi study to identify high-priority research, action, and advocacy needs. Taken together, these three approaches (Fig. 1.1) led us to propose a research agenda to accelerate improvements in QoC.

We begin with an introduction on the importance of QoC in reducing unmet need for FP and of accelerating progress on improving QoC in this chapter, followed by review of frameworks on QoC in health and FP in Chap. 2. The MoHFW has begun implementing a National Quality Assurance Programme, which has set QA standards and assesses and scores facilities on key performance indicators. These then become the basis for facilities to take actions to remedy deficiencies. Recently there has been increased emphasis on FP programming based on the rights framework which includes QoC. The trend is to see QoC not just as leading to desirable FP outcomes but as a right of clients. The rights consideration broadens the attributes of SRH information, education, and services to include availability, accessibility, and acceptability in addition to quality. Building on the foundation of QoC, it also includes accountability of the programme, a more active role of the community, and enhanced agency and autonomy of the clients. Based on the rights framework, understanding of factors influencing continuation of contraceptive use, and QI efforts, the chapter proposes a more comprehensive framework of variables that need to be influenced to improve QoC. It proposes that health systems and community environments could play an enabling, motivating, and empowering role

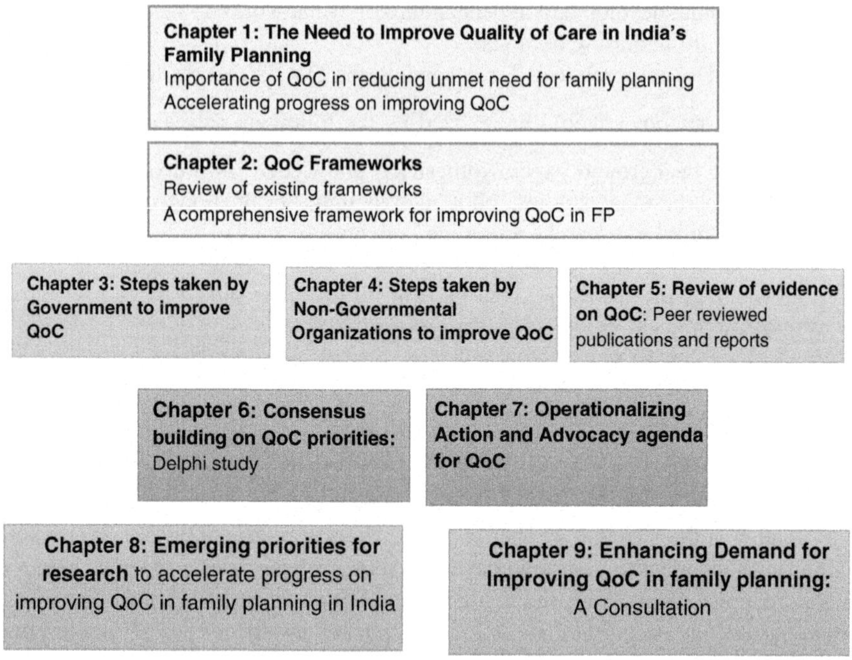

Chapter 1: The Need to Improve Quality of Care in India's Family Planning
Importance of QoC in reducing unmet need for family planning
Accelerating progress on improving QoC

Chapter 2: QoC Frameworks
Review of existing frameworks
A comprehensive framework for improving QoC in FP

Chapter 3: Steps taken by Government to improve QoC

Chapter 4: Steps taken by Non-Governmental Organizations to improve QoC

Chapter 5: Review of evidence on QoC: Peer reviewed publications and reports

Chapter 6: Consensus building on QoC priorities: Delphi study

Chapter 7: Operationalizing Action and Advocacy agenda for QoC

Chapter 8: Emerging priorities for research to accelerate progress on improving QoC in family planning in India

Chapter 9: Enhancing Demand for Improving QoC in family planning: A Consultation

Fig. 1.1 A schematic of the background paper (prepared by the authors)

for both providers to provide and clients to demand QoC, and provide an ecosystem for sustained improvement.

Government, private sector, and non-governmental organizations (NGOs) have taken several steps to improve QoC. In Chap. 3, we first briefly describe measures implemented by government to improve QoC. Many NGOs and donors are assisting government to improve QoC by strengthening systems, implementing comprehensive interventions, and improving provider competencies for delivering specific contraceptive methods. In Chap. 4 we discuss standalone interventions implemented by NGOs for service delivery of DMPA and IUCD, and for reaching young people with requisite QoC. The private sector has two major operational modalities—social franchising and social marketing—to expand the basket of choice and services, provide quality information and care, and use commercial and non-commercial distribution networks to make the subsidized commodities available to the target population. Although many steps have been taken for QA to improve QoC in both of these modalities, continuous progress on QA and QI is needed.

We discuss peer-reviewed and other published research studies on QoC in FP in India in Chap. 5. In 1994, the ICPD was organized in Cairo, and this conference upheld the principle of "reproductive rights". Central to the conference resolutions was the concept of voluntary, informed choice of contraception and the importance of providing information and services to all individuals and couples. Therefore, we begin our review of research studies from 1995. We discuss the studies under four categories:

1.5 Approach for Developing Background Paper

1. *Status of QoC*: what is the QoC delivered
2. *Interventions*: evaluations of interventions and their scale-up
3. *Factors affecting QoC*: provides deeper understanding which may lead to formulating innovative interventions
4. *Assessing consequences*: benefits and costs of different levels of QoC.

A research study, however, might address one or more of the above.

As mentioned earlier, we found very few peer-reviewed studies during the last two decades in India on QoC in FP. As a recent global review on FP is available (Askew and Brady 2013), we compare our findings with its conclusion on QoC in FP and find that there is good concordance between the two.

In Chap. 6, we discuss the findings of the Delphi study. After consultations with key informants and based on our review, we prepared a list of 29 research, 6 action, and 3 advocacy agenda questions. In the first round, the participants rated each question as high, medium, or low priority. These were scored as 3, 2, and 1, respectively, for pooling the responses. This led to the identification of high-priority questions. Middle-priority questions formed the basis for the second round, in which participants ranked the questions in order of priority. High-priority questions in the first round and the highly ranked questions in the second round led to a list of key questions that should be addressed by a research agenda.

Chapter 7 looks at operationalizing the action agenda and advocacy processes that may be considered based upon past experiences, to strengthen commitment. The Delphi study identified three priority actions: activating QoC organizational mechanisms; enhancing accountability of the programme; and improving supply. This chapter discusses what may be needed to operationalize this prioritized action agenda. There is a general perception that commitment to QoC among key stakeholders needs to be strengthened. Advocacy to strengthen such commitment to QoC is critical.

We bring together the findings from actions taken to improve QoC (Chaps. 3 and 4) using the framework developed (Chap. 2), review of research studies (Chap. 5), and the results of the Delphi study (Chap. 6), as well as the need for research to support a prioritized action agenda and processes for advocacy (Chap. 7), in order to develop a proposed research agenda in Chap. 8. Each research question is further discussed and a possible research approach to addressing that question is presented. We conclude with a summary of research issues that need to be addressed to accelerate improvements in QoC in FP in India. Thus, this background paper provides a roadmap for researches that will support evidence-based actions to accelerate improvements in QoC in India.

In the last chapter, we present a summary of a consultation held in January 2017 on enhancing the demand for QoC in FP in India. All available evidence indicates that QoC is only improving gradually. Compared to interventions and research to increase the capacity of the service delivery system to provide QoC, there are very few interventions that focus on enhancing demand for quality. Issues affecting QoC extend beyond the service provider setting, influencing clients before they arrive to seek services. Important determinants that affect demand for QoC include the client's agency and autonomy, gender norms, socio-cultural factors, costs of seeking quality care, myths and misconceptions about methods, and access. Clients' perspectives on the services they receive are an essential part of understanding and assessing QoC, and these are shaped by cultural values and norms, past experiences, perceptions of the role of the health system, and interactions with providers.

There are several opportunities for improving QoC. Socio-economic status, particularly of women, is gradually improving. The information and communication revolution offers an opportunity to empower clients and communities to enhance demand for QoC. The trade-off between increasing access and improving quality is shifting in favour of quality. The consultation held in Jodhpur during 16–17 January 2017 focused on enhancing demand for QoC to further the ongoing discussion on QoC in FP, and contributed ideas to build the discourse around this important issue in the country. The participants shared perspectives on enhancing demand for QoC in FP in India. This consultation helped gather new perspectives and understandings of key issues in improving QoC. Sub-streams of work to take forward this discourse to address important issues are identified.

References

Achyut, P., Nanda, P., Khan, N., & Verma, R. (2014). *Quality of care in provision of female sterilization and IUD services: An assessment study in Bihar*. New Delhi: International Center for Research on Women.

Ali, M. M., Cleland, J., & Iqbal, S. (2012). *Causes and consequences of contraceptive discontinuation: Evidence from 60 demographic and health surveys*. Geneva: World Health Organization.

Askew, I., & Brady, M. (2013). *Reviewing the evidence and identifying gaps in family planning research: The unfinished agenda to meet FP2020 goals*. Background document for the Family Planning Research Donor Meeting, Washington, D.C., December 3–4, 2012. New York: Population Council.

Black, R. E., Levin, C., Walker, N., Chou, D., Liu, L., & Temmerman, M. (2016). Reproductive, maternal, newborn, and child health: Key messages from disease control priorities 3rd edition. *Lancet*. http://dx.doi.org/10.1016/S0140-6736(16)00738-8.

FP2020. (2014). *FP2020 principles of rights and empowerment*. http://www.familyplanning2020.org/images/content/documents/FP2020_Statement_of_Principles_FINAL.pdf. Accessed July 30, 2017.

Jain, A. K. (1989). Fertility reduction and the quality of family planning service. *Studies in Family Planning, 20*(1), 1–16.

Jain, A. K., Obare, F., Rama Rao, S., & Askew, I. (2013). Reducing unmet need by supporting women with met need. *International Perspectives on Sexual and Reproductive Health, 39*(3), 133–141. https://doi.org/10.1363/3913313.

MoHFW (Ministry of Health and Family Welfare). (2007–2008). *District level household and facility survey-4, 2007–2008*. Mumbai: International Institute for Population Sciences.

MoHFW (Ministry of Health and Family Welfare). (2012–2013). *District level household and facility survey-4, 2012–2013*. Mumbai: International Institute for Population Sciences.

MoHFW (Ministry of Health and Family Welfare). (2014). *India's vision FP 2020*. New Delhi: Family Planning Division, Government of India.

References

MoHFW (Ministry of Health and Family Welfare). (2016). *India observes health week to promote healthy living.* https://www.nhp.gov.in/india-observes-health-week-to-promote-healthy-living_pg. Accessed February 16, 2018.

NFHS-3 (National Family Health Survey-3). (2005–2006). International Institute for Population Sciences, Mumbai.

NFHS-4 (National Family Health Survey-4). (2014–2015). International Institute for Population Sciences, Mumbai.

PFI (Population Foundation of India). (2014). *Robbed of choice and dignity: Indian women dead after mass sterilization.* http://populationfoundation.in/files/fileattached/Fileattached-1480404258-Report-on-Bilaspur-Visit-2-December-2014.pdf. Accessed January 14, 2018.

Sedgh, G., Ashford, L. S., & Hussain, R. (2016). *Unmet need for contraception in developing countries: Examining women's reasons for not using a method.* New York: Guttmacher Institute.

Chapter 2
What is Quality? Quality of Care Frameworks

Abstract In this chapter, we present a review of existing frameworks and a comprehensive framework for improving quality of care in family planning. We discuss the two most popularly used frameworks for defining quality of care: Donabedian's framework in health (Donabedian, 1988), and the Bruce-Jain framework in family planning. Then we briefly describe the National Quality Assurance Programme of the Ministry of Health and Family Welfare (MoHFW), Government of India, implemented by the National Health Systems Resource Centre (NHSRC). We discuss how the Bruce-Jain quality of care framework relates to rights-based programmes. We conclude the chapter with a discussion of what we can learn regarding quality of care in family planning from quality of care improvement in the health sector. Finally, more recent literature discusses the importance of health system functioning and community norms in a programme's ability to provide quality of care, in essence providing an ecosystem for quality of care improvement interventions to achieve their full potential. Building on this literature, we present a comprehensive framework for improving quality of care.

Keywords Quality of care frameworks · Quality assurance · Ecosystem
Health system

2.1 Donabedian's Quality of Care Framework

The earliest and most widely used framework for QoC in the health sector was offered by Donabedian. He described a framework in 1966 for assessing QoC that was flexible enough to apply to many situations, and refined it over a period of two decades. Figure 2.1 illustrates the framework relating structure, process, and outcomes. Structures of health care are defined as the physical and organizational aspects of care settings, which include facilities, equipment, personnel, and operational and financial processes supporting medical care. The processes of health care are performed in order to improve patient health in terms of promoting

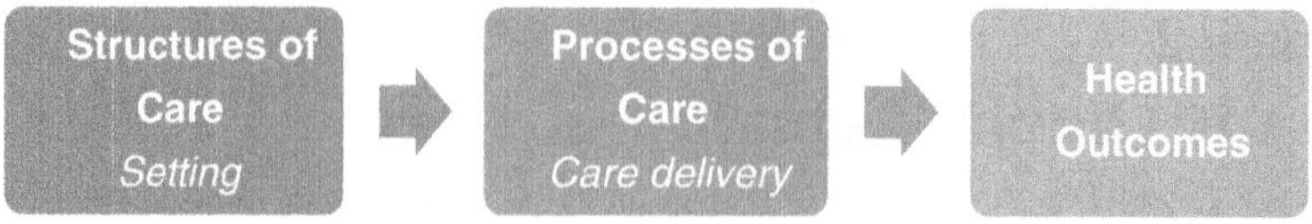

Fig. 2.1 Donabedian's quality of care framework *Source* Framework for assessing the quality of medical care. Reprinted with permission from Donabedian A: Evaluating the quality of medical care

recovery and functional restoration to achieve the health outcomes of survival and patient satisfaction.

Donabedian's framework does not explicitly consider patients' connect in terms of economic or social factors outside of the care delivery system (McDonald et al. 2007). He states:

> This is justified by the assumption that one is interested … in whether what is now known to be "good" medical care has been applied. Judgments are based on considerations such as the appropriateness, completeness and redundancy of information obtained through clinical history, physical examination and diagnostic tests; justification of diagnosis and therapy; technical competence in the performance of diagnostic and therapeutic procedures, including surgery; evidence of preventive management in health and illness; coordination and continuity of care; acceptability of care to the recipient and so on.

Donabedian had included effectiveness, efficiency, and equity as dimensions of QoC (Singh et al. 2015). Maxwell (1984) explicitly included patient-centredness as a dimension of QoC. The UK government's framework (1997) included patient satisfaction as an indicator of patient-centredness. The Council of Europe expanded the dimensions of QoC to include all the above five features. The WHO (2015) has developed a universal framework for QoC that can be applied across multiple health programmes. The framework includes the following characteristics:

- *Safe*: delivering health care which minimizes risks and harms to service users, including avoiding preventable injuries and reducing medical errors.
- *Effective*: providing services based on scientific knowledge and evidence-based guidelines (health outcomes, efficacy, technical competence, supporting services, follow-up/continuity, functional infrastructure).
- *Timely*: reducing delays in providing/receiving services.
- *Efficient*: delivering health care in a manner which maximizes resource use and avoids wastage (cost, avoidance of waste).
- *Equitable*: delivering health care which does not vary in quality because of personal characteristics such as gender, race, ethnicity, geographic location, or socio-economic status (access, availability, choice, utilization).
- *People-centred*: providing care which takes into account the preferences and aspirations of individual service users and the cultures of their communities (respect, information, satisfaction, acceptability).

In 2001, the Institute of Medicine prepared a report titled *Crossing the Quality Chasm: A New Health System for the 21st Century*, which includes all the above dimensions but also focuses on fostering innovations in health care to improve

2.1 Donabedian's Quality of Care Framework

QoC. The Joint Commission on Accreditation of Health Care Organizations has developed a framework for QoC that is to serve as a basis for accreditation. It largely focuses on the supply side to include effectiveness, efficiency, and safety, but also includes the dimensions of access and availability for measuring equity.

Thus, improved QoC increases the likelihood of desired individual and facility-level health, coverage of key practices, and people-centred outcomes. Based upon a functional health system ("structure" in the Donabedian framework), the process of QoC is seen as comprising the following:

- *Provision of care*: evidence-based practices in care, actionable information system, and functional referral system.
- *Experience of care*: effective communication, respect and dignity, and emotional support.

These need to be supported by competent and motivated human resources as well as essential physical resources.

2.2 Quality Improvement in the Health Sector

In 2015, the Bill and Melinda Gates Foundation organized a seminar (BMGF and Duke University 2015) to review innovative experiences in improving QoC in the health sector, with particular attention to RMNCH+A. A review of the seminar deliberations provides a good opportunity to discuss the latest innovative efforts to improve QoC. Broadly, these innovations dealt with measurement and improvement of quality, although almost all interventions to improve quality also included some measurement efforts.

2.2.1 Measurement of Quality

The purpose of measuring quality could be QI, QA, or policy and planning. The purpose would determine which criteria should be used to select indicators.

A major difficulty in routinely measuring quality is the amount of effort required. Structural variables are relatively easier to measure compared to both process and/ or outcome variables. However, it is important to measure process as well as to look at outcome measures over time. A comprehensive approach would be to create a dashboard with a parsimonious set of critical variables. The data quality need to be improved, while data also needs to be used for strategic purposes, including for improving counselling.

Methodology for measuring QoC uses QA indicators, including for the accreditation of facilities as well as for establishing quality standards and providing a seal of QoC. The tools for measurement of quality include the following:

During provision of services	For ensuring preparedness	For demanding quality through voice
• Quality of care toolkit • Checklists, mentors, coaches • Training, protocols, supplies • Clinical guidelines, history taking • Quality improvement process, nurse/ doctor mentor • Clinical reviews	• Provider preparedness (competencies, inventory) • Health system readiness (health system pillars, problem solving, self-assessment)	• Role of Panchayats • Client/ Community factors, feedback

Fig. 2.2 Interventions to improve quality *Source* Framework for assessing the quality of medical care. Reprinted with permission from Donabedian A: Evaluating the quality of medical care

- facility walk-through; facility audits
- observation; case sheets, tests, objective, structured clinical examinations
- interview of clients, providers, and managers; exit interviews
- self-assessment
- mobile monitor
- use of standardized patients.

2.2.2 Quality Improvement

A major issue in QI is the relative emphasis to be placed on structure and process variables (Fig. 2.2). In case performance contracts are issued, one needs to consider carefully whether contracts should be input based or output based.

As mentioned earlier, many improvement processes also include measurement and feedback. Although the above learning about measurement and improvement of quality of services also applies to service provision for FP, several important considerations for QoC in FP do not figure in it. For instance, informed choice of methods is an important consideration for QoC in FP, which does not find any mention in these innovations. Similarly, the role of information provision is inadequately emphasized. Finally, a constellation of services is not systematically considered.

2.3 Reproductive, Maternal, Newborn, Child, and Adolescent Health: Strategy and Quality of Care

The RMNCH+A approach was launched by MoHFW in 2013 (MoHFW 2013) to address the major causes of mortality among women and children as well as delays in accessing and utilizing health care and services. The RMNCH+A strategic approach uses the concept of "continuum of care" for a life-cycle approach. It includes priority interventions for each thematic area. It also introduces new initiatives, like the use of the scorecard to track performance, the National Iron-Plus Initiative to address the issue of anaemia across all age groups, and comprehensive screening and early interventions for defects at birth, diseases, and deficiencies among children and adolescents. Family planning is seen as one of the critical components of the RMNCH+A strategy.

The bottleneck analysis for interventions identified lack of focus on improving quality of service delivery along with low quality of training and skill building, among others. The strategy argues that provision of quality services requires an efficient organization of work and a high level of motivation and consciousness about quality, besides the addition of infrastructure and human resources, equipment, drugs, and supplies. It emphasizes the importance of ensuring affordability and the elimination of social barriers and processes that lead to exclusion of the poor and marginalized.

The MoHFW had established QA mechanisms for sterilization services extending up to the district level, following directions from the Supreme Court in 2005. The RMNCH+A strategy extended the scope of the QA system to include the full range of RMNCH+A services.

The organizational arrangements for QA include: (1) the Central Quality Supervisory Committee; (2) state QA committees, QA cells, and full-time quality assessors; (3) district QA committees, QA cells, and QA officers; and (4) quality circles at the district hospital level. Subsequently, a National Quality Assurance Programme (NQAP) was established, housed at the NHSRC.

2.4 National Quality Assurance Programme

The MoHFW wanted to start an accreditation programme for its facilities at the district and sub-district levels (Jhalani 2014). It examined available accreditation frameworks—Indian Public Health Standards (IPHS) (MoHFW 2012), the National Accreditation Board for Hospitals, the International Organization for Standardization—in terms of the following criteria: specificity to public health, systems approach, inbuilt certification, flexibility to customize, sustainability and scalability, and low cost of implementation. The MoHFW found these frameworks deficient on one or more of these criteria. Therefore, it decided to launch the NQAP.

The NQAP has set QA standards and assesses and scores facilities on key performance indicators. Through this process, facilities will be accredited. The process will be implemented by an organizational structure at the national, state, district, and facility levels. Continuous internal assessment is done at the hospital level; district QA units will undertake quarterly assessments; state QA units will perform periodic assessment and provide state-level certification, and the NHSRC will issue national-level certification.

Quality assurance standards have been established in the following eight areas with specifics for each public health programme, including FP:

- *Service provision*: availability of curative services; availability of RMNCH+A services; provides diagnostic services.
- *Patient rights*: information about available services and modalities; sensitive to gender/religion/culture; no barriers to physical access, language; privacy, confidentiality, and dignity; informing and involving patients and their families/informed consent; no financial barriers to access.
- *Inputs*: availability of infrastructure that meets prevalent norms; ensuring physical safety of infrastructure; programmes for fire safety and other disasters; adequate trained staff; provision of drugs and consumables; availability of equipment and instruments.
- *Support services*: inspection, testing, and calibration of equipment; procedures for storage, etc.; safe, secure, and comfortable environment for patients, staff, etc.; procedures for upkeep and maintenance of facility; 24 × 7 water and power backup; clean linen for patients; compliance with statutory and regulatory requirements; defined roles and responsibilities; procedure for monitoring quality of outsourced services.
- *Clinical services*: procedures for registration, admission, clinical assessment and reassessment, continuity of care, nursing care, antenatal care, FP; procedures for identifying high-risk and vulnerable cases; following of standard guidelines; procedures for safe drug administration; procedures for updating clinical records; procedures for discharge, emergency services, diagnostics, anaesthesia, surgical, end-of-life care/death.
- *Infection control*: prevention/measurement of hospital infections; procedure for hand washing and asepsis; standard practices and materials for protection; processing of equipment and instruments; ensuring infection prevention—layout, environmental care; handling of biomedical and hazardous waste.
- *Quality management*: patient and employee satisfaction measurement; internal and external QA; standard operating procedure for all supporting services; mapping of processes and making them efficient; internal audit; defined quality policy and quality objectives; seeking continued improvement.
- *Outcome*: productivity with established benchmarks; efficiency; care and safety; service quality indicators.

Detailed guidelines comprising checklists have been prepared for assessment. Some incentives have been linked with performance and certification. The NQAP is being rolled out over a few years to cover all facilities, beginning with district hospitals.

2.5 Quality of Care Frameworks for Family Planning

Family planning differs from health or medical care in that it largely addresses the needs of healthy individuals for SRH information and services. Germain (2014) argues:

> The people who use or potentially use SRH information and services are generally healthy and in the prime of their life. They have the right to control what happens to their bodies, to have control over their sexuality, including their sexual and reproductive health, and to have access to and use of SRH services, education and information without any form of discrimination, violence or coercion by any source, including their families, health care providers and policymakers.

In this context, FP programmes not only need to serve married women; unmarried women and adolescent girls must also receive attention.

Although FP services are generally provided in the context of health services and include both clinical and non-clinical contraception, the development of frameworks for QoC in FP has proceeded in different directions than those for health care. Building on Donabedian, Jain (1989) proposed facility readiness and the process of providing services as determining the quality of FP services.

The issue of QoC in FP and RH programmes gained worldwide prominence in the 1990s with the Bruce-Jain framework on QoC. It defined quality as the "way individuals are treated by the system providing services" (Bruce 1990; Jain 1989). The framework identifies six elements, which apply mainly to clinical services, relevant to improving QoC in FP programmes:

- *Choice of contraceptive methods*: This element refers to the number of contraceptive methods offered on a regular and reliable basis. Clients who have more contraceptive options to choose from are more likely to find a method which meets their needs.
- *Information given to clients*: Clients who receive clear, accurate, unbiased information tailored to their needs are more likely to be satisfied with the method of their choice.
- *Interpersonal relationships*: This element refers to relationships between provider and client which are built on respect, positive rapport, trust, and cultural and gender sensitivity. Good interpersonal relationships and effective interpersonal communication between health care provider and patient are important for improving patient satisfaction, treatment compliance, and health outcomes.
- *Technical competence*: This element refers to provider knowledge and skills, and adherence to good clinical practices and standard operating procedures.
- *Continuity and follow-up*: High-quality services should provide some mechanism for follow-up with FP clients in order to address the client's concerns, manage side effects, provide guidance on issues of adherence, and facilitate method switching or discontinuation (in cases where method switching is provider dependent).

Structure/Program readiness	Process/QoC	Outcome/impact
• Contraceptives and supplies • Facilities and equipment • Staff training and attitudes including technical competency • IEC materials • Supervision and management	• Choice of methods • Information exchange • Interpersonal exchanges • Best technical practices • Mechanisms to encourage continuity • Appropriate constellation of services	• Client knowledge • Client satisfaction • Client health • Contraceptive acceptance and continuation • Contraceptive prevalence • Total fertility rate

Fig. 2.3 Bruce-Jain framework related to Donabedian's framework *Source* Framework for assessing the quality of medical care. Reprinted with permission from Donabedian A: Evaluating the quality of medical care

- *Appropriate constellation of services*: Because women often view FP as closely related to other reproductive and child health needs, integration of FP into services such as postpartum services, post-abortion care, and child health services may provide further opportunities for reaching women who otherwise may not seek FP services.

Figure 2.3 shows how the Bruce-Jain framework can be related to the Donabedian framework.

To date, the Bruce-Jain framework is the most widely used framework in assessing and improving QoC in FP, although some elements may receive more emphasis than others in this process.

Quality of care is a multidimensional issue that may be defined differently by different stakeholders:

- Clients generally perceive QoC as the way they are treated, whether their needs are met and their concerns addressed.
- Providers often see QoC as comprising the technical dimensions of services provided, including effectiveness and safety.
- Programme managers may focus on management systems including logistics, supplies, human resources, supervision and monitoring.
- Policy makers are often concerned with cost, efficiency, and health outcomes as well as equity.

2.6 Rights of Clients and Providers

The International Planned Parenthood Federation (IPPF) promotes good QoC by ensuring that clients have the right to information, access to services, choice, safety, privacy and confidentiality, dignity and comfort, and continuity of services and opinion. To fulfil clients' rights, the needs of service providers must be met as well. These needs include: training, information, infrastructure and supplies, guidance, respect and encouragement, feedback, and opportunities for self-expression.

The IPPF has recently revised its QoC framework guided by the vision of "enabl[ing] all people to act freely on their sexual and reproductive health and rights by providing quality SRH services" (Fig. 2.4). Besides the rights of the clients and needs of the providers, its guiding principles and values include human rights, dignity, equity, social inclusiveness, accountability, and freedom from stigma. It seeks to direct special attention to youth, gender, and underserved, vulnerable, and marginalized populations. Espousing a client-centred approach, the framework specifies the following six inputs: safe and confidential environment; secured supply chain; comprehensive integrated services; adequate financial resources; well-managed services; effective communication and feedback systems; and highly skilled and respectful personnel.

2.7 Quality of Care as a Right of Clients

The trend is to see QoC not just as leading to desirable FP outcomes but as a right of clients. The ICPD Programme of Action 1994 mandates that SRH policies and programmes respect, promote, and fulfil human rights, particularly of women and adolescents (Germain 2014). Two sets of human rights can be considered, as follows. The first set of human rights helps to create an enabling environment emphasizing gender equality and empowerment of women. The second set of rights focuses on access to the means to secure and maintain SRH. The Programme of Action requires promotion and protection of human rights and fundamental freedoms, as well as adherence to medical and public health ethics and technical standards in the delivery of SRH services, education, and information. Quality of care, therefore, needs to operationalize a second set of rights, that is, human rights norms, for the quality of SRH information, education, and services.

The rights considerations broaden the attributes of SRH information, education, and services to include availability, accessibility, and acceptability in addition to quality. Germain (2014) argues that the following six action elements, building on Bruce's six elements, are necessary to achieve quality that meets human rights norms:

1. Widest possible range of choices among contraceptive methods
2. Decent facilities, equipment, and commodities
3. Training and supervision of service providers
4. Essential package of integrated SRH services
5. Outreach and communication
6. QA mechanisms (monitoring, redress for individuals, and mechanisms to remedy policy failures as well as prevent and correct discrimination in access and other abuses).

Vision		
To enable all people to act freely on their sexual and reproductive health and rights by providing quality sexual and reproductive health services.		
Guiding Principle and Values		
International Planned Parenthood Quality of Care Charter Rights of the Clients, Needs of the Providers	Human rights Diversity Equity	Social inclusion Accountability Stigmafree
Cross Cutting Themes		
Youth	Gender	Underserved, vulnerable and marginalized
Key Elements		
Client-Centered Approach		
Safe & Confidential Environment	Appropriate set-up/structure • Accessible location • Safe environment for both providers and clients • Privacy and confidential	Secured Supply Chain Management System	Commodity security • Durable, high quality and appropriate equipment • Logistics management • Range of contraceptive methods
Comprehensive Integrated Services	Wide range of SRH services • Comprehensive information • Client follow-up • Reliable referral system and follow-up • Evidence based service delivery • Informed client decision-making and consent	Adequate Financial Resources	Financial sustainability • Diverse sources of income • Costed services • Fee system including ner refusal policy • Resource allocation for QoC • Good financial management system
Well-Managed Services	Efficient service delivery approach • Effective supportive supervision • Provider self-assessment • Performance driven culture • Policies, standard operating procedures, guidelines • Client-driven demand for service delivery • Clinical governance	Effective Communication & Feedback Systems	Strong monitoring and evaluation system • Quality improvements based on data • Access to comprehensibl information • Community support/buy in • Assessment mechanisms • Client empowered to take an active part in the care process • Community participation
Highly Skilled and Respectful Personnel		Sufficient and appropriat number of staff and functions • Supported and motivated staff • Technically competent	**Staff** committed to providing high quality services • Interpersonal skills • Client-focused personnel

Source: Quality of Care Framework, 2015. International Planned Parenthood Federation

Fig. 2.4 IPPF's framework on quality of care (IPPF 2015)

2.7 Quality of Care as a Right of Clients

Thus, the inclusion of human rights considerations broadens QoC to the functioning of the whole programme. Hardee et al. (2014) provides a framework for voluntary programmes that respect, protect, and fulfil human rights (Rodriguez et al. 2013). This would require inputs and activities at policy, service, community, and individual levels, as Fig. 2.5 shows. The outputs of such programmes are envisaged to be the following:

- FP services are available, accessible, acceptable, and of the highest quality (according to the Bruce framework)
- Accountability systems are in place
- The community actively participates in programme design, monitoring, accountability, and QI
- Community norms support health and rights
- The agency of individuals is increased.

Thus, programmes can build on the bedrock of QoC to add each of these points to incorporate human rights considerations (see Fig. 2.6).

Using a health and human rights rationale, WHO guidelines on ensuring human rights in the provision of contraceptive information and services suggest the addition of the following elements to informed decision making and quality of contraceptive information and services in Bruce's six elements of QoC:

- Accessibility including non-discrimination, availability, and acceptability of contraceptive information and services
- Privacy and confidentiality
- Participation of clients
- Accountability of providers to clients.

To advance consideration of human rights, WHO and the United Nations Population Fund (WHO and UNFPA 2015) have developed implementation guidelines. The programme categories for this purpose include ensuring access for all; commodities, logistics, and procurement; organization of health facilities; outreach and integration; QoC; participation of clients and accountability to clients. In addition, comprehensive sexuality education and humanitarian contexts are highlighted.

A key challenge is how to best support health care providers and programme managers to ensure that they use human rights aspects in provision of contraceptive services. For this purpose, WHO has developed checklists to ensure that health care providers and managers adhere to these aspects. A view is emerging in the literature that QoC and human rights are two intrinsically connected approaches; realization of one without the other is not possible.

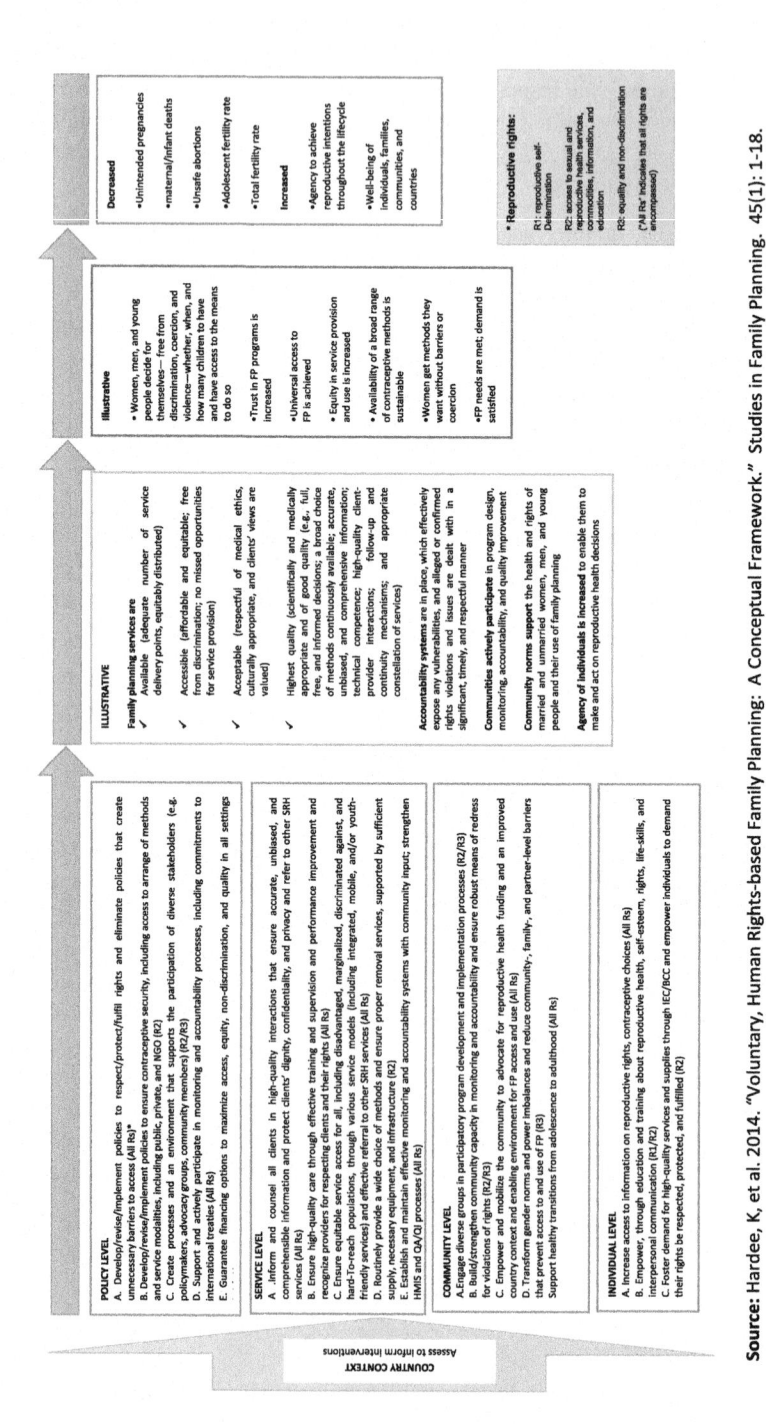

Fig. 2.5 Framework for voluntary family planning programmes that respect, protect, and fulfil human rights (Hardee et al. 2014)

Source: Hardee, K, et al. 2014. "Voluntary, Human Rights-based Family Planning: A Conceptual Framework." Studies in Family Planning. 45(1): 1-18.

```
We see quality of care as a continuum from leading to desired outcomes to fulfilling individual rights
                                    ↓
              Leading to desired family planning outcomes
                                    ↓
        Accessible, available, acceptable, affordable family planning services
                                    ↓
                   Available to clients and communities
                                    ↓
       Community norms support health and rights and community actively participates
                                    ↓
                        Individual aegncy is achieved
```

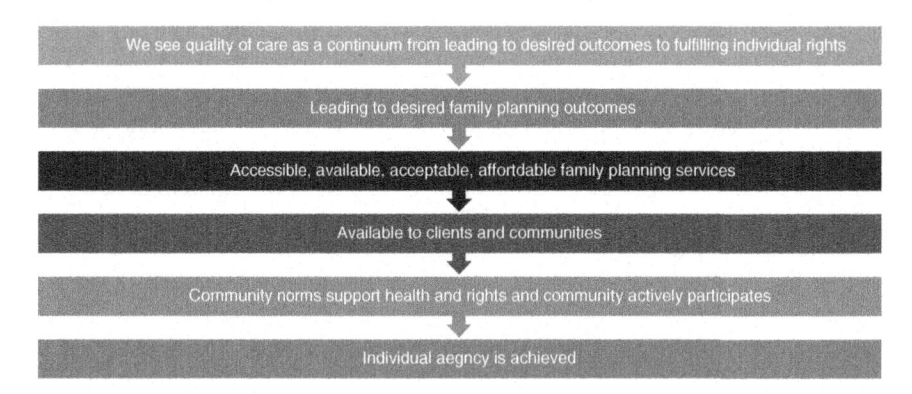

Fig. 2.6 Quality of care to rights-based approach *Source* Framework for assessing the quality of medical care. Reprinted with permission from Donabedian A: Evaluating the quality of medical care

2.8 Incorporating Health System and Community Influences in Quality of Care Framework

One of the significant outcomes of QoC in FP services is to reduce discontinuation of the use of a contraceptive method because of method-related reasons. This phenomenon, called contraceptive discontinuation, is defined as starting contraceptive use and then stopping for any reason while still at risk of an unintended pregnancy.

Castle and Askew (2015) review the reasons, challenges, and solutions for contraceptive discontinuation. Analyses of demographic and health survey data indicate that 38% of women with an unmet need for modern contraception have used a modern method of contraception in the past but have chosen to discontinue use.

On average, over one-third of women who start using a modern contraceptive method stop using within the first year, and over one-half stop before two years. More than half of discontinuations are among women experiencing contraceptive failure or having method-related problems with its use, and so are still in need of effective contraception to prevent an unintended pregnancy.

Demographic and health survey data indicate that between 7 and 27% of women stop using a contraceptive method for reasons related to the service environment, including service quality, availability of a sufficient choice of methods, commodity stock-outs, and ineffective referral mechanisms. Jain and colleagues have termed discontinuation as the "leaking bucket" that reduces the impact of FP programmes (Jain 2014).

Programmatic strategies to reduce discontinuation include improving service quality. The quality of FP services has also been shown to have a direct impact on whether a woman continues, discontinues, or switches a method. For example, Blanc et al. (2002) analysed QoC using the Family Planning Programme Effort score and found that between 7 and 27% of women stopped using contraception for reasons related to low quality of the service environment, and that between 40 and 60% of the overall discontinuation rate reflects decisions based on QoC. The authors conclude that, as contraceptive use increases, FP programmes would benefit from a shift in emphasis from primarily reaching out to new clients, towards greater investment in reducing discontinuation rates. This conclusion is supported by the analyses of Jain et al. (2013) described above. The challenge, therefore, is determining how programmes can enhance QoC so that women's rights are met and discontinuation is reduced.

A review of the literature reveals few examples of QI interventions that have been evaluated explicitly in terms of impact on discontinuation. Jain et al. (2014) summarize this evidence, including simulations and cross-sectional and longitudinal studies. Some quasi-experimental studies that tested interventions to improve QoC and continuity of use have failed to demonstrate a substantial effect of the interventions. RamaRao and Mohanam (2003) suggest that research has not adequately determined whether particular aspects of service quality (for example, counselling, method choice, provider–client interactions, information including improved knowledge about physiology) are more likely to influence continued use, either singly or in combination. For example, the evaluation in the Philippines (Jain et al. 2012) found that although women receiving higher QoC were more likely to continue using contraception after three years, and to report fewer unintended pregnancies and unwanted births, the provider training intervention itself did not have a direct effect on continuation, even though it did improve provider knowledge and provider–client interactions. The authors propose that this is because other contextual and logistical factors, as well as the socio-cultural environment, may also have influenced the QoC received, such as method choice, access, rates, and cost. Thus, although it is unlikely that a single element of QoC will influence continuation, investments that improve the multiple elements of service quality may have the desired impact. As Jain et al. (2014) say:

> The issue is not only about adding methods to the contraceptive mix in a country or improving the quality of counselling per se. Rather it is about meeting women's reproductive health needs, their right to have a choice among contraceptive methods, their right to make informed choices, and their right to receive accurate information from service providers about the method they select and about switching methods whenever the initial one is no longer suitable.

Castle and Askew (2015) propose a theory of change that identifies several pathways through which interventions addressing health systems, service quality, and the socio-cultural environment could reduce unnecessary discontinuation. Health system elements include elimination of stock-outs, offering an adequate method mix, sufficiently trained and oriented human resources, and access to services assured through multiple service delivery options and supportive policy environment. Service quality elements include comprehensive and balanced counselling, full information about switching, elimination of provider bias, respectful treatment of clients, systematic management of clients coming late for resupply, and appropriate engagement of male partners. The socio-cultural understanding includes the meaning and interpretation of side effects and misconceptions as well as intentionality, motivation, and ambivalence. These would support continuation and support restart and switching for discontinuers.

Castle and Askew propose implementation research, intervention testing of specific approaches through quasi-experimental studies, and social science research.

Quest Project uses a conceptual framework that explicitly seeks to understand the effect of health systems and influencing environment on QoC received by clients. The health system includes strategic vision; voice and participation; transparency and accountability; responsiveness of institutions; effectiveness and efficiency; intelligence and information; and ethics. The influencing environment includes agency and autonomy; equity and non-discrimination; values and community norms; and political and legal context (ibid.).

In a recent work, Jain (2017), based on the comparison of quality across frameworks, past experiences, and issues faced in measuring quality, recommends modifications to the QoC framework. The availability of a method is reflected by the availability of commodities, equipment, and a provider competent in offering that method. The element of constellation of services is retained, and technical competence is broadened to include competency in providing the method chosen, compliance with infection prevention practices, and information exchange with clients. The component of information given to clients is replaced by information exchange consisting of information solicited from clients to ensure the selection of a method appropriate to the client's needs, preferences, and circumstances, information given to clients to ensure effective contraceptive use, and information given to clients to ensure continuity of care and contraceptive use. The element of interpersonal relations explicitly includes the treatment of clients with dignity and respect, and ensuring their privacy and confidentiality.

Most programmes to improve QoC recognize the role of the environment as enabling in nature. For instance, the SEED programme of EngenderHealth considers the following elements in an enabling environment: policy, programme, and community environment, coupled with social and gender norms, the support functions of health systems, and facilitation of healthy behaviours.

2.9 A Proposed Comprehensive Framework for Interventions to Improve Quality of Care

Based on the rights framework, the understanding of continuation, and QI efforts, we hypothesize that health systems and community environments could play an enabling, motivating, and empowering role for both providers and clients (Fig. 2.7). Variables having an influence on QoC can be categorized as having an immediate, proximate, or a distal effect directly or indirectly (Table 2.1).

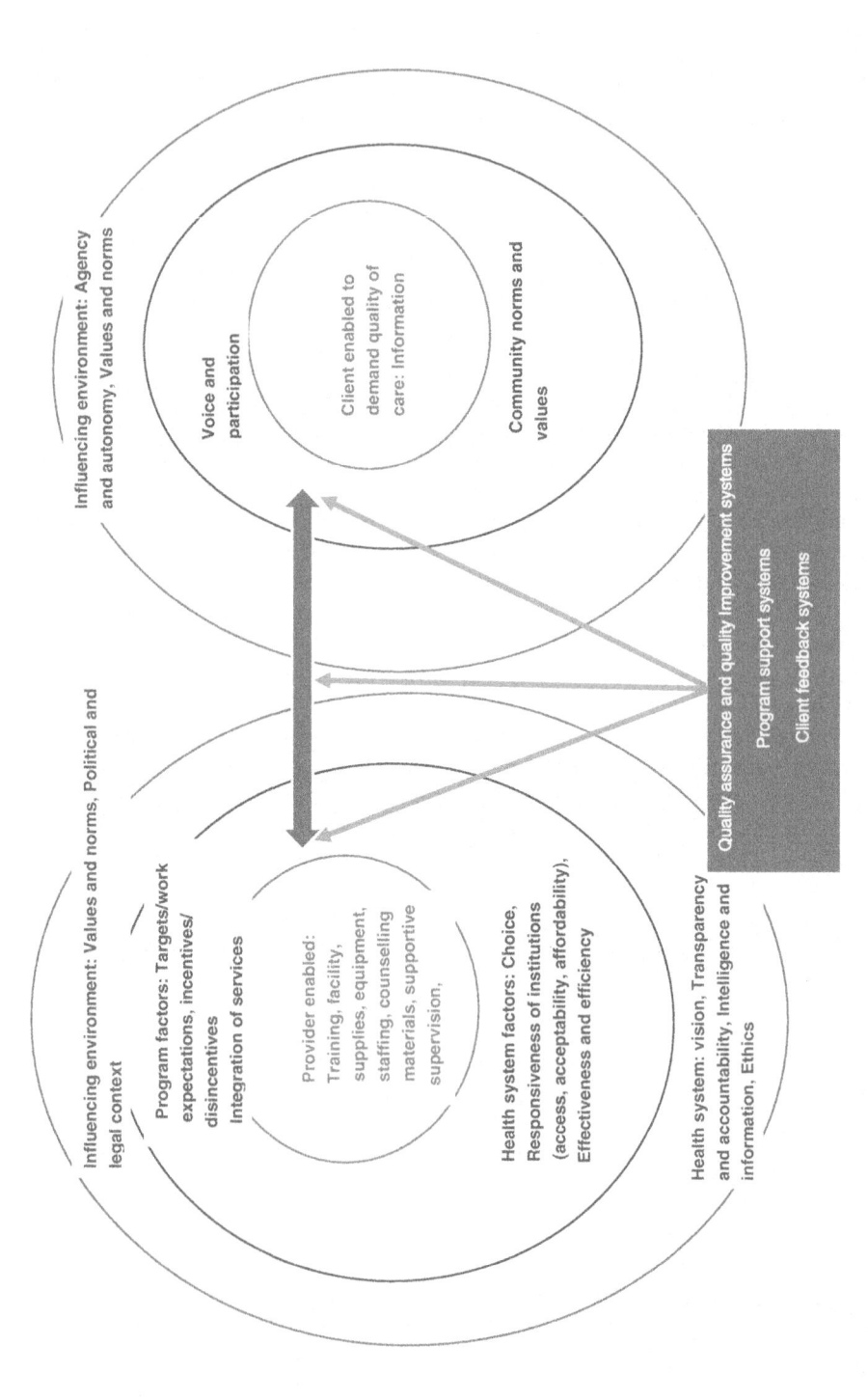

Fig. 2.7 Improving quality of care: systems framework *Source* Framework for assessing the quality of medical care. Reprinted with permission from Donabedian A: Evaluating the quality of medical care

2.9 A Proposed Comprehensive Framework for Interventions ...

Table 2.1 Variables to be influenced to improve quality of care *Source* Framework for assessing the quality of medical care. Reprinted with permission from Donabedian A: Evaluating the quality of medical care.

	Immediate	Proximate	Distal
Direct	Competencies of providers (training, mentoring), facility, staffing, supplies, equipment, counselling materials, job aides, supportive supervision Client enabled to demand QoC: information to clients	Targets/work expectations, incentives to users, incentives to facilitators, incentives/disincentives to providers and programme officials Integration of services Voice and participation	Influencing environment for providers: values and norms Influencing environment for clients: agency and autonomy, community values and norms
Indirect	QA and QI systems Programme support systems (budgeting, planning, monitoring, etc.) Client feedback	Health systems: choice available to clients, responsiveness of institutions (access, availability, acceptability, affordability), effectiveness, and efficiency Community norms and values	Influencing environment: political and legal context Health system: strategic vision, transparency and accountability, intelligence and information, ethics

We will use this framework to review actions taken to improve QoC (Chaps. 3 and 4), research studies (Chap. 5), and the Delphi study in Chap. 6. Health systems and community environment provide an ecosystem for important efforts to improve QoC in FP.

References

Blanc, S. K., Curtis, S. L., & Croft, T. N. (2002). Monitoring contraceptive continuation: Links to fertility outcomes and quality of care. *Studies in Family Planning, 33*(2), 127–140.

BMGF (Bill & Melinda Gates Foundation), & Duke University. (2015). Workshop on *Quality of health care: Measurement and efforts to improve quality*. Neemrana Fort-Palace, 30 June–1 July.

Bruce, J. (1990). Fundamental elements of the quality of care: A simple framework. *Studies in Family Planning, 21*(2), 61–91.

Castle, S., & Askew, I. (2015, December). *Contraceptive discontinuation: Reasons, challenges, and solutions*. New York: Population Council.

Department of Health. (1997). The new NHS: modern, dependable. https://www.gov.uk/government/publications/the-new-nhs

Donabedian, A. (1988). The quality of care: How can it be assessed? *JAMA, 121*(11), 1145–1150. https://doi.org/10.1001/jama.1988.03410120089033.

Germain A. (2014). Discussion note for the ICPD beyond 2014 conference on human rights: Meeting human rights norms for the quality of sexual and reproductive health information and services. In *ICPD Beyond 2014 Expert Meeting on Women's Health: Rights, Empowerment and Social Determinants*. 30 September–2 October 2013, Mexico City. Background paper 2b. https://www.unfpa.org/sites/default/files/resource-pdf/Human_Rights.pdf Accessed on April 5, 2018

Hardee, K., Kumar, J., Newman, K., Bakamjian, L., Harris, S., Rodríguez, M., et al. (2014). Voluntary, human rights-based family planning: A conceptual framework. *Studies in Family Planning, 45*(1), 1–18.

http://pai.org/quest-project/. Accessed October 7, 2016.

http://sites.duke.edu/healthqualityworkshop/workshop-summary/. Accessed July 20, 2016.

http://www.ema.europa.eu/ema/index.jsp?curl=pages/partners_and_networks/general/general_content_000574.jsp&mid=WC0b01ac0580789733. Accessed September 12, 2016.

https://www.engenderhealth.org/our-work/seed/. Accessed October 7, 2016.

https://www.jointcommission.org/achievethegoldseal.aspx. Accessed September 12, 2016.

http://www.nrhmhp.gov.in/sites/default/files/files/Iron%20plus%20initiative%20for%206%20months%20-5%20years.pdf. Accessed September 12, 2016.

IPPF (International Planned Parenthood Federation). (2015). *Quality of care framework 2015*. London: IPPF.

Jain, A. (2014). *The leaking bucket phenomenon in family planning*. Champions for Choice, September 9. https://champions4choice.org/2014/09/the-leaking-bucket-phenomenon-in-family-planning/. Accessed January 19, 2018.

Jain, A. (2017). *Quality of care in the context of rights-based family planning*. New York: Policy brief, Population Council.

Jain, A. K. (1989). Fertility reduction and the quality of family planning services. *Studies in Family Planning, 20*(1), 1–16.

Jain, A. K., Ramarao, S., Kim, J., & Costello, M. (2012). Evaluation of an intervention to improve quality of care in family planning programme in the Philippines. *Journal of Biosocial Science, 44*(1), 27–41. https://doi.org/10.1017/S0021932011000460.

Jhalani, M. (2014). *National quality assurance programme*. Presentation made during the NHSRC Convention, 2014.

Maxwell, R. J. (1984). Quality assessment in health. *British Medical Journal of Clinical Research and Education, 288,* 1470–1472.

McDonald, K. M., Sundaram, V., Bravata, D. M., Lewis, R., Lin, N., Kraft, S. A., et al. (2007, June). *Closing the quality gap: A critical analysis of quality improvement strategies* (Vol. 7: Care coordination). Technical reviews, No. 9.7. Agency for Healthcare Research and Quality.

MoHFW (Ministry of Health and Family Welfare). (2012). *Indian public health standards: Guidelines for community health centres*. New Delhi: Directorate General of Health Services, Ministry of Health and Family Welfare, Government of India.

MoHFW (Ministry of Health and Family Welfare). (2013, July). *A strategic approach to reproductive, maternal, new-born, child and adolescent health (RMNCH+A) in India*.

RamaRao, S., & Mohanam, R. (2003). The quality of family planning programs: Concepts, measurements, interventions, and effects. *Studies in Family Planning, 34*(4), 227–248.

Rodriguez, M., Harris, S., Willson, K., & Hardee, K. (2013). *Voluntary family planning programs that respect, protect, and fulfill human rights: A systematic review of evidence*. Washington, D. C.: Futures Group.

Satia, J., Chauhan, K., (2015). Urban Health Initiative (UHI): A comprehensive intervention to address family planning needs of the urban poor in Uttar Pradesh. In J. Satia, K. Chauhan, A.

Bhattacharya, & N. Mishra (Eds.), *Innovations in family planning: Case studies from India*. New Delhi: SAGE.

Singh, S., Krishnan, A., & Kaushal, K. (2015). *Landscape of QoC in India*. Amaltas Research and Development Consulting. New Delhi.

WHO (World Health Organization). (2015). *Improving the quality of care for reproductive, maternal, neonatal, child and adolescent health in South-East Asia Region*. Geneva: WHO.

WHO (World Health Organization), & UNFPA (United Nations Population Fund). (2015). *Ensuring human rights in contraceptive service delivery: Implementation guide*. Geneva: WHO, New York: UNFPA.

Chapter 3
Steps Taken by the Government of India to Improve Quality of Care

Abstract This chapter discusses the measures implemented by government to improve quality of care. It also presents the efforts, supported by NGOs and donors, at assisting government to improve its quality of care by improving systems, implementing comprehensive interventions, and improving provider competencies for delivering specific contraceptive methods. To ensure quality of family planning services, efforts led by the government include introducing guidelines for equipment, supplies, infrastructure, outreach strategies, human resources, and establishing quality assurance committees at state and district levels. To address the concern over quality of sterilization services, specifically at camp facilities, the Family Planning Indemnity Scheme was introduced. In order to improve the method mix and offer more choices to couples, the Ministry of Health and Family Welfare is expanding the basket of contraceptive products by introducing new methods and improving the supply chain logistics management information system. Several NGOs with support from various donor agencies are working with government to augment service delivery to improve quality of care. This has resulted in increased acceptance of contraceptive methods, indicating some impact of improved quality of care.

Keywords Family planning indemnity scheme · Supply chain
Logistics management · Technical assistance

3.1 Guidelines Developed by the Government of India to Ensure Quality in Family Planning Service Delivery

The MoHFW of the Government of India has introduced measures to ensure quality of FP services, which include setting up standards and guidelines for equipment, supplies, infrastructure, outreach and communication strategies, human resources, and ensuring quality care in FP services by establishing QA committees (QACs) at state and district levels (MoHFW 2013).

To provide technical guidance to health facilities at various levels, the first edition of a manual on standards in sterilization was developed in 1989. This manual was revised in 1996, 1999, and 2006. The first manual on QA was published in 1996, and a revised version was released in 2006.

Indian Public Health Standards (IPHS) guidelines were launched in the year 2005, and later revised in 2012. The IPHS lays down norms for physical infrastructure, services (essential and desirable), human resources, equipment, drugs, and diagnostics at public health facilities. However, there is no inbuilt system of quality certification under the IPHS (MoHFW 2012).

After the orders of the Hon'ble Supreme Court of India in 2005 (Supreme Court, 2005), the government has prepared manuals for service delivery of each contraceptive method and has established structures for QA by introducing norms for ensuring uniformity with regard to sterilization procedures. The order more specifically recommends:

1. Creating a panel of doctors and health facilities for provision of sterilization services
2. Establishing criteria for empanelment of doctors for conducting sterilization procedures
3. Developing a checklist to be followed by every doctor before carrying out sterilization procedures
4. A uniform pro forma for obtaining consent of the person undergoing sterilization
5. Setting up of QACs for ensuring enforcement of pre- and post-operative guidelines regarding sterilization procedures.

Quality assurance guidelines have been developed by MoHFW for planning a spectrum of services provided at public health facilities. The guidelines define processes for implementing QA in the states, and in turn states are required to meet the minimum standards defined in the guidelines. *Operational Guidelines for Quality Assurance in Public Health Facilities* and the accompanying volumes of "Assessment Tools" released by MoHFW in 2013 have been prepared for health services in the arena of RMNCH+A and various disease control programmes. The guidelines list eight areas of concern: (*a*) service provision; (*b*) patient rights; (*c*) inputs; (*d*) support services; (*e*) clinical services; (*f*) infection control; (*g*) quality management; and (*h*) outcome. Each area of concern has standards and measurable elements against which the facility is assessed. The manual on *Quality Standards for Urban Primary Health Centres* (MoHFW 2015) has 35 standards under 8 areas of concern with 198 measurable elements (ME). For example:

Area of Concern: Clinical Services

Maternal and child health standards

Standard E21 The facility has established procedures for abortion and family planning as per government guidelines and law.

ME E21.1 Family planning counselling services provided as per guideline.

ME E21.2 The facility provides spacing method of family planning as per guideline.

ME E21.3 The facility provides limiting method of family planning as per guideline.

Area of Concern: E Clinical Services

Standard E7 Facility has established procedure for family planning as per government guideline.

ME E7.1 Family planning counselling services provided as per guidelines.

ME E7.2 Facility provides spacing method of family planning as per guideline.

ME E7.3 The facility provides IUCD service for family planning as per guidelines.

ME E7.4 Facility provides counselling services for medical termination of pregnancy as per guidelines.

ME E7.5 Facility provides abortion services for 1st trimester as per guideline.

A separate checklist for FP has been designed with intent to assess the availability, accessibility, utilization, and quality of FP services delivered at the primary health centres (PHCs). Counselling constitutes the major portion of the checklist. The checklist has checkpoints related to contraceptives (condoms, OCPs, POP, emergency contraceptives), IUCD, safe abortion services (primary management of spontaneous abortions, medical termination of pregnancy using manual vacuum aspiration, medical abortions). Assessment of FP services is combined with assessment of general clinic, dressing room, and emergency.

The list of technical and operational guidelines developed by MoHFW for augmenting FP quality and services is as follows:

- *Quality Assurance Manual for Sterilization Services*
- *Standards for Female and Male Sterilization Services*
- *IUCD Reference Manual for Medical Officers and Nursing Personnel*
- Reference manual on contraception
- *Manual for Family Planning Insurance Scheme*
- Revised Compensation Package to Acceptors of IUD Insertions and Sterilization at Public Health Facilities and Private Accredited Health Facilities
- Check List for Monitoring of Family Planning Services in the State/District
- Permission for Procurement of NSV Kits through NHM Flexipool at State/District Level
- Permission for Procurement of IUCD Kits through NHM Flexipool at State/District Level
- Guidelines for Repositioning IUCD
- Revised Budget Guidelines for Camps in Sterilization Services
- Fixed-Day Static Services for Sterilization—Operational Guidelines
- Standard Operating Procedures for Sterilization Services in Camps
- Guidelines for Administration of Emergency Contraceptive Pills by Health Care Providers
- Guidelines for Clinical Skill Building Training in Male and Female Sterilization Services
- Guidelines for Home Delivery of Contraceptives (Condoms, OCPs, and ECPs) by ASHA at the doorstep of beneficiaries.

3.2 Family Planning Indemnity Scheme

To address the concern over the quality of sterilization services, specifically at camp facilities, the Family Planning Insurance Scheme was introduced by MoHFW in 2005, which was renamed the Family Planning Indemnity Scheme in 2013. The second edition of the scheme was released in 2016 (MoHFW 2016a). This is an effort to address the complications, failures, and deaths following sterilization procedures. Under this scheme, states/union territories would financially compensate by making payment of claims to acceptors of sterilization in the event of death or complications following sterilization. The scheme is implemented by budgeting it through the respective state/union territory programme implementation plans (PIPs). The MoHFW has carried out state-level workshops to disseminate manuals and guidelines in all states as well as divisional workshops in high-priority states. At the state level, a five-member state indemnity subcommittee from within the state quality assurance committee (SQAC) has the responsibility to redress, dispose, and disburse claims/complaints received through the district quality assurance committee (DQAC), to the district health society as per the procedure and time frame laid down in this manual. At the district level, a five-member district indemnity sub-committee from within the DQAC reviews and processes the claims received.

3.3 Quality Assurance Committees

For strengthening QA activities, QACs are formed at the national level (the Central Quality Supervisory Committee), the state level (SQAC, the state QA unit, and QA assessors [empanelled]), the district level (DQAC, the district quality assurance unit), and the district hospital level (district quality team). Specific roles and responsibilities are defined for each level to ensure that the standards for female and male sterilization as laid down by the government are followed in respect of pre-operative measures (pathological tests) and operational facilities (sufficient numbers of the necessary equipment, aseptic condition, and post-operative follow-ups).

The QACs are expected to conduct medical audit of all sterilization-related deaths and for sending reports to the SQAC. The committee is expected to collect information on all hospitalization cases related to complications following sterilization, as well as sterilization failure. It is mandated to review sterilization services for QoC at all static institutions (i.e., government and accredited private providers) as per the standards, and to recommend remedial actions for institutions not adhering to standards. The DQAC reviews, reports, and processes compensation claims for onward submission to the SQAC under the National Family Planning Indemnity Scheme.

3.4 Expanding Contraceptive Choice and Improving Access

To improve the method mix and offer more choices to couples, the MoHFW repositioned IUCD in 2006. This was supported by community mobilization efforts, capacity building of service providers, intensive demand creation, and awareness generation activities. Special emphasis was placed on PPFP services with the introduction of PPIUCD. Introduction of DMPA, POPs, and Saheli (the weekly pill) was also being rolled out in 2016. To improve access and availability, fixed-day quality services are operationalized at community health centres (CHCs) and higher levels for providing quality FP services. Quality services in hard-to-reach areas are sought to be provided by mobile teams for improving access to sterilization services, along with accreditation of more private/NGO facilities to increase the provider base for FP services under public–private partnership (PPP). The counselling experience is sought to be improved through the appointment of RMNCH+A counsellors at district hospitals and other high-volume facilities.

The MoHFW is piloting the RH commodities logistics management information system (RHCLMIS), successfully pilot-tested in Odisha, in other states to improve contraceptives supply management up to peripheral facilities. Capacity enhancement initiatives are being held by conducting on-site training through dedicated mobile training teams.

On the demand side, awareness generation activities in the form of development of new audiovisual software, display of posters, billboards, and other materials are being developed. In 2016, during the National Family Planning Summit held in New Delhi, the MoHFW released a new 360-degree communication campaign for increasing awareness regarding FP by placing maternal and child health (MCH) and well-being at the centre of the approach (MoHFW 2016c). The new strategy focuses on the role of various stakeholders such as the mother, father, mother-in-law, and husband as well as the role of community health workers, doctors, nurses, auxiliary nurse midwives (ANMs), and ASHAs to educate and inform couples about the benefits of FP for the health of mother and child.

3.5 Improving Quality of Care in Government Service Delivery with Support from NGOs and Development Partners

3.5.1 Strengthening Systems

Strengthening systems is one of the avenues for improving QoC in government services. The UNFPA has supported the Government of Maharashtra in strengthening its QA system following MoHFW guidelines, and the Government of Odisha in improving its RHCLMIS.

3.5.1.1 Quality of Care Through Quality Assurance Systems: The Government of Maharashtra Experience

The UNFPA has been supporting the Government of Maharashtra in improving QoC at its facilities to provide improved FP services (Satia 2015). A pilot project for QA was implemented in 2006–2007 in Ahmednagar district, where QA checklists were used in selected health facilities with encouraging results. The feasibility and usefulness of the intervention were proven, and the state decided to scale up the intervention in six districts. This led to the setting up of district QA cells in subsequent years, followed by the creation of structures for monitoring and review. The intervention consists of visits to each facility once in a quarter by members of the district quality assurance group (DQAG) to identify actions needed to improve quality by utilizing the checklist. In 2011, the effort was scaled up to cover 12 districts. All CHCs/SDH (Sub-divisional Hospitals) and 24 × 7 PHCs (about 75 in a district) were covered, and an additional six districts were included in 2012.

The first phase of QA system implementation was evaluated in 2012. The evaluation compared the performance on the checklist of the facilities under the QA system to other comparable facilities not in the QA system in the same and neighbouring districts. The average assessment score for QA facilities was significantly higher than non–QA facilities, and the QA facilities scored higher than non–QA facilities on almost all sections of the QA checklist. The evaluator recommended that more attention was needed on output indicators and that, along with QA, other barriers to improving output including appropriate staffing and demand creation also needed to be addressed to realize the full potential of QA efforts. Subsequently, the Government of Maharashtra has decided to extend the intervention to the entire state to institutionalize a system of assessment of QoC in RH services at public health institutions and to improve it through systematic actions taken by the health system.

Several other states have made efforts to operationalize a QA system. For instance, Odisha promotes quality in FP services through orientation and activation of DQACs for conducting facility audits and client exit interviews. However, evidence suggests that the functioning of the system among states is highly variable (Nanda et al. 2010).

3.5.1.2 Reproductive Health Commodities Logistics Management Information System: Streamlining the Supply Chain for Contraceptives in Odisha

A continuous and adequate supply of contraceptives along with an enabling environment and efficient service delivery mechanism are prerequisites for successful implementation of a FP programme. To increase voluntary access and utilization of FP services, the Directorate of Family Welfare, Government of Odisha, formulated strategies for improved FP efforts in the field, regular monitoring, information management and dissemination, and streamlining the contraceptive logistics and supply system. The RHCLMIS, a multi-tier logistics management information system for contraceptives, was introduced. The system is supported by a web and SMS-based application which helps in managing the supply and demand of contraceptives delivered through the government at district, block and sub-centre levels. The system deals with collection, processing, and reporting of logistics-related data at different levels and provides instant access to contraceptive stock information and pipeline status by tracking supply and stock at all levels. This was needed not just to provide services and contraceptive security to people, but also to ensure QoC in implementation at various operational levels in the health system. Regular checks are done to ensure quality control through testing of product samples at government-authorized quality testing laboratories. There have been no stock-outs of contraceptives since the system became operational. Improved availability of contraceptive supplies enables informed choice (Chauhan 2015b).

3.5.2 Public–Private Collaboration for Comprehensive Improvement of Quality of Care in Government Services

Several NGOs with support from various donor agencies are working with government to augment service delivery to improve QoC. We discuss three of them below—Ananya in Bihar, the Urban Health Initiative (UHI) in Uttar Pradesh, and Karuna Trust in Karnataka. They have taken several steps to improve QoC comprehensively in government programmes and to supplement the government's IEC activities.

3.5.2.1 Ananya: An Integrated Approach to Achieve Health for All

Ananya was conceived as a coordinated, complementary set of interventions in Bihar to enhance the provision of health services including FP, and to shape demand for them. The programme was implemented in partnership with the Government of Bihar in 8 focal districts and 64 blocks for a period of five years (2011–2015). The districts were Patna, Samastipur, Begusarai, Khagaria, Gopalganj, East Champaran, West Champaran, and Saharsa. Innovations under the programme aimed to address demand-side outcomes, namely, knowledge, attitudes, and practices related to maternal and newborn health, including FP (with a focus on postpartum use of intrauterine devices [IUDs] and tubal ligation); the supply-side indicators related to availability and quality at the facility level (Mishra and Bishnoi 2015).

Improving QoC at the Facility Level Counselling corners were established in public facilities; supportive supervision was strengthened; staff were trained using on-site training by mobile nurse trainers and mini skill labs; and evidence-based tools and approaches were promoted that ensure sustained improvements in FP service. CARE introduced self-driven facility assessment tools and QI processes for health facilities on different parameters like supplies, procedures, and equipment. These assessments help to address shortcomings in functioning like unavailability of IUDs, OCPs, Nischay kits, etc., and also the shortage of skilled service providers. At the facility level, a QI process has been introduced in coordination with the QA cell of the Department of Health and Family Welfare and other partners. The QI team, consisting of one person from each department of the facility, meets monthly to review the progress of QI efforts and to plan for the next month. Team members include a labour room nurse, the block health manager, the medical officer in charge, a pharmacist, a data entry operator, an administrator, and custodial staff. The team assesses and prioritizes the needs of its facility, sets short-term goals to address these needs, identifies steps to achieve each goal, and designates an individual who is responsible for each step. With regard to the technical interventions in FP, CARE has focused on integrated antenatal and postpartum counselling and referrals.

IUCD Mobile Van Camps The camps were held at the health sub-centre/PHC/anganwadi centre or panchayat community centre with two scheduled visits per block/village in a month. The services were provided by two trained nurses, one of them examining the women using the pregnancy test, the Nischay kit, and the other performing the IUD insertion. Quality being the focal point, an average of four clients were served per hour, using a no-touch technique. A toll-free number was provided to the clients in case of any queries or complications faced.

Social Franchising In addition, through social franchising, qualified private providers were utilized. The choice of methods was expanded through provision of DMPA in collaboration with Abt Associates.

Field-Level Workers To improve the functioning of field-level workers, different mediums were used, like paper-based tools and job aids, pre-decided content for monthly health sub-centre meetings, reference materials for communication, and standard operating procedures for overall improvement of the field-level worker's ability to deliver timely, appropriate, and high-quality services.

Continuum of Care Services This project was piloted in Saharsa district from July 2011 to December 2013 to test the coverage and quality of services by field-level workers using information and communication technology tools (mobile phone) compared to paper-based tools. With its application design by Dimagi and multimedia job aids by BBC WST, the pilot included features like schedulers, checklists, and due lists for continuum of care, which were thoroughly pre-tested by the field-level workers. Use of mobile phones was pilot-tested to improve the communication skills of ASHAs including mobile Kunji as well as Kilkari. Monitoring, learning, and evaluation are a part of cross-cutting solutions where data is collected using the Lot Quality Assurance Survey and direct observation of delivery methodology.

3.5.2.2 Urban Health Initiative: A Comprehensive Intervention to Address Family Planning Needs of the Urban Poor in Uttar Pradesh

The UHI programme framework was aligned with the FP programme goal of the Government of India and Government of Uttar Pradesh (Satia and Chauhan 2015). The overall goal was to increase contraceptive use as a key intervention to reduce maternal and infant mortality and implement evidence-based strategies which are aligned with government schemes and programmes so that they are more likely to be replicated and scaled up to benefit greater numbers of people. This effort aimed to increase contraceptive use in the urban slums of 11 cities of Uttar Pradesh, including four core cities and seven cities where the programme was scaled up. Urban slums are categorized as large, family-size, clustered temporary housing, with appalling health and sanitation conditions and poor access to quality health services. Programme strategies were directed towards improving supply of services and QoC to enhance access to FP information, counselling, methods, and supplies as well as increasing demand through BCC and community mobilization. This has resulted in increased utilization of services and supplies by couples as well as a higher contraceptive prevalence rate, including use of modern contraceptives and long-acting and permanent methods. Quality of care was improved in service delivery through the following measures:

Quality Fixed Services Days In line with the government's fixed static day approach, UHI worked with both government and private facilities to ensure that key FP services were assured on an identified day and time per week or month at an expected stable price or free of cost. This package is meant to expand people's access to quality services, and is delivered by skilled and licensed doctors and nurses having adequate equipment and supplies. It also includes payment to the clients and community workers, as often people seeking services are accompanied by urban ASHAs and/or their supervisors who help people in uptake of services. It also supports either contracted-in or trained counsellors at high-volume facilities to improve counselling.

Clinical Training, Whole Site Training, and Mentoring of Providers This was carried out for adherence to assured standards of practice in both government and identified private providers. The UHI trained a large number of service providers and outreach workers on QoC and counselling. Clinic-based workers were trained in infection prevention. All service providers were oriented with technical updates and government guidelines. They were supported by toolkits and job aids as well as IEC material.

Private Sector Involvement with QoC Nearly 60% of deliveries are estimated to be taking place in private facilities. Therefore, UHI decided to increase private sector involvement in FP. Non-governmental organizations provided a list of private providers to which clients were generally referred and which were conveniently accessible. A UHI team visited these facilities to assess their ability and willingness to provide the desired quality of services. The clinics ensure QoC including infection prevention. The initiative also expanded choice of methods by introducing DMPA in private facilities.

Strengthening Women's Groups Women's groups were strengthened in order to share their experiences and need for quality services and to engage them in planning and implementing actions to benefit their community.

Data for Monitoring, Mentoring, and Motivating Data for monitoring, mentoring, and motivating was used for continuous improvements in quality and new acceptors, including in divisional and state-level reviews. The Service Delivery Point Survey included facility audits and provider interviews at select health facilities, audits of selected pharmacies and outlets, and exit interviews with FP and maternal, newborn, and child health clients at high-volume facilities. The client exit interviews helped identify women's reasons for their FP or maternal or child health visit, the types of services received, counselling practices, and general perceptions of QoC. The pharmacy audit was undertaken in about 100 pharmacies in each study city, and a brief audit was undertaken with registered medical providers and retail outlets within the communities where women live.

3.5.2.3 Repositioning Family Planning: Strengthening Services Within the Primary Health Care Centre in Karnataka by Karuna Trust

Karuna Trust, with support from the PFI, is managing government PHCs in Karnataka (Chauhan 2015a). The project covers a population of 313,500 served by 64 sub-centres under 14 PHCs in 12 districts of Karnataka. The main objective of this effort is to encourage couples to delay the first pregnancy and promote spacing between pregnancies. The initiative has sought to improve the quality of reproductive and child health and primary health care programmes through accreditation by the National Accreditation Board for Hospitals and Health care Providers, and continuous review and monitoring mechanisms. It has used interventions at the structure, process, and outcome levels to improve QoC, including:

Building a Skilled, Motivated Workforce This seeks to enable doctors, nurses, managers, and providers to deliver quality FP and RH services. The capacity of the staff of the 14 PHCs is being enhanced with training in management, counselling, BCC, and IEC skills. Training of service providers is undertaken at regular intervals. This includes training of medical officers and staff nurses on various contraceptive methods (injectable, IUCDs) and orientation on adolescent health issues. Further, ASHAs and ANMs are taught counselling techniques to encourage the use of FP methods. "Training of trainers" sessions are organized and qualified personnel are used for carrying out the refresher trainings. The Block health education officers, senior male health workers, and other PHC staff are specifically trained on conducting IEC/BCC activities to encourage community participation and acceptance of FP methods of the user's own choice.

Orientation of Community Members This is undertaken at regular intervals. Community members are trained to take an active part in the VHNSCs and self-help groups by involvement in planning and monitoring activities on the ground.

Improving Management Medical officers, administrators, and supervisors at the PHCs are oriented on management and QA methods through the preparation of standard operating protocols and patient feedback mechanisms. Regular meetings of the Arogya Kalyan Samitis (health welfare committees) have enhanced the quality of service provision.

Continuous Review and Monitoring Mechanism Participatory rapid appraisal provides an understanding of service capabilities at the health facilities in terms of availability, access, and quality. Outcomes are monitored over time.

3.5.3 *Improving Provider Competence for Intrauterine Contraceptive Devices and Non-scalpel Vasectomy*

Non-governmental organizations have supported the government in strengthening the competency of providers: the Johns Hopkins Program for International Education in Gynecology and Obstetrics (JHPIEGO) through training for PPIUCD and interval IUCD services, EngenderHealth for NSV, and Ipas through on-site training for IUCD services. They have reported increased acceptance of these methods, indicating some impact of improved QoC.

3.5.3.1 Training for IUCD by JHPIEGO

Implemented by the MoHFW, Government of India, with technical support from JHPIEGO, this initiative aims to increase substantially the use of IUCD as an FP method. This effort has been developed as a competency-based clinical training approach that is rapidly scalable and easily adaptable within the government system (Kumar et al. 2014). A six-day training course on IUCD insertion (CuT 380A) using a mix of clinical and pedagogic approaches was developed. Clinical competencies were to be built through repeated practice of IUCD insertion using the Zoe model. As a result of this intervention, replication of the training programme was achieved by 9 of 12 intervention states in four months and in all states within six months. Standard training protocols and checklists for monitoring training quality as well as trainee performance are in place. It is expected that IUD services will be provided at static facilities by providers trained by these trainers.

Training increases the technical knowledge and counselling skills of providers with regard to IUD and quality of services. To assess the quality of counselling and services provided before, during, and after insertion of the IUD, 10 IUD users from each PHC were interviewed. The proportion of IUD users who reported the quality of IUD services received to be good (score of 25 or more out of 34) increased from 26 to 73%. Further improvement could also be achieved by providing continuous supportive supervision and a positive programmatic environment where the provision of good-quality services and services for IUD are valued.

In the case of postpartum provision of IUCD (PPIUCD), a standard learning resource package, a PPIUCD insertion video, and other job aids, skills checklists, and facility-based IEC materials were developed. The training was to update the knowledge and skills of the service providers and trainers for providing quality PPIUCD services to women delivering at the health facilities, initially at the district hospitals and medical colleges. The training was followed by supportive supervision at the health facility to help the institutions initiate quality PPFP services.

The training approach used competency-based training of trainers and service providers. Both doctors and nurses were taught performance improvement measures based on standards-based management and recognition, and there were post-training supportive supervision visits to the facilities. To improve the quality of counselling, dedicated FP counsellors were provided at each intervention facility, which facilitated the uptake of PPFP and PPIUCD services. Standard training protocols and checklists for monitoring training quality as well as trainee performance are in place, ensuring high-quality training and post-training follow-up, and emphasizing quality of services including infection prevention practices, training management, and monitoring.

3.5.3.2 On-site Training Model for Comprehensive Abortion Care in India: A New Approach

Comprehensive abortion care (CAC) is an integral component of maternal health interventions under the NHM. The Government of India, as part of its commitment to strengthening women-centred CAC services, especially in the public sector, has taken various initiatives including standardization of CAC training and service delivery, which began with the launch of the national *Comprehensive Abortion Care Training and Service Delivery Guidelines* in 2010. These guidelines were instrumental in transforming abortion care from a purely medical approach to a woman-centred CAC approach, and in simplifying service provision within the context of the law (MoHFW 2016b).

The Ipas Development Foundation has been working in close collaboration with the MoHFW of the Government of India to strengthen the programme in 13 states for effective implementation of the safe abortion component. Increasing access to CAC services at national and state levels, based on the context and current interventions, would require a renewed focus on appropriate technologies for CAC service delivery, especially medical methods of abortion, prioritization of strategies for strengthening CAC services, and identification of innovative strategies for strengthening CAC services.

The CAC effort was pilot-tested as an on-site training model, as compared to centralized training, covering 186 providers. On-site training has advantages in terms of addressing site-specific barriers, preparing a critical mass of providers, and providing ongoing mentoring after training, as well as having a follow-up mechanism for client feedback. A mobile training team carried out site strengthening, skill building, and community intermediary engagement. On-site post-training support included clinical mentoring, client follow-up and continuous education, as well as administrative and logistics support. The training was highly successful in reducing provider myths and biases, increasing PPIUCD acceptors five-fold, effecting a seven-fold increase in the number of providers offering services, and creating a more balanced contraceptive method mix. While the on-site training model offers potential for scale-up, it is costlier compared to centralized training.

In 2014, CAC guidelines were further strengthened through the release of the national CAC training package. The Government of India has since taken the initiative to establish model centres to demonstrate the ideal set-up for CAC training and service delivery. It aims to improve the quality of woman-centred CAC training and subsequent CAC service provision. Training centres in eight states—Bihar, Chhattisgarh, Maharashtra, Madhya Pradesh, Karnataka, Rajasthan, Jharkhand, and Assam—have been selected in phase I of the initiative. These centres will be used to establish highest-quality parameters in various aspects of CAC, including privacy and confidentiality; equipment and supplies; infection prevention; use of safe technologies; documentation and reporting, etc.

3.6 Other Efforts to Improve Quality of Care

There have been several pilot projects to improve QoC. Some of them are briefly described below.

3.6.1 EngenderHealth: Improving Quality at Service Sites Through Quality Circles (COPE)

The COPE model (client-oriented, provider-efficient) (EngenderHealth 2003) aims to improve quality through increased communication between staff and supervisors via the "facilitative supervision" approach, monitoring health services to identify gaps in standards and practice, and addressing the diverse learning needs of health care staff at a facility through whole-site training. The COPE model is a pioneering set of tools for health providers and other staff to continuously assess and improve quality of services. Instruction manuals and online courses in infection prevention are made available. Site staff uses quality measuring tool annually and supervisors determine whether clients' rights are being upheld and staff needs are being met.

The cost analysis tool measures the cost of providing health services and can be used to improve the efficiency of staff.

Community COPE (EngenderHealth 2005) is a participatory process that builds partnership between health care staff and community members to make health services more responsive to local needs.

In Uttar Pradesh, a QI pilot was launched in June 2002 under the Innovations in Family Planning Services (IFPS) Project, with the aim of establishing approaches to address these issues. The intervention, developed with technical assistance from EngenderHealth, was piloted mainly at the block level at 18 sites in two districts, Sitapur and Saharanpur. A marked improvement was reported in service quality standards between baseline and the first quarterly assessment in both pilot districts, in both quality-certified and non-certified sites. Progress was found to be less dramatic in subsequent quarters, but the initial improvements were sustained throughout the project period. Of the 18 pilot sites, 9 were certified as quality sites and received the Gold Star Logo.

A review of the COPE-based action plans showed that approximately 30% of the problems identified by staff were effectively solved within days and an additional 40% in subsequent months. Client exit interviews revealed a general satisfaction with the quality of services following the QI project. It was observed that provider experience in site management and service provision showed a marked improvement at all of the QI sites. Providers reported better coordination among site staff, improved supervision, and greater accountability. Further, joint problem solving and teamwork led to improved staff interaction. Staff reported treating clients with more respect, and giving due regard to informed choice and confidentiality. Increases in service utilization were registered across almost all services, but there was considerable variation in the extent of increases. Relative to the baseline, the increase in the number of outpatients was 99%, and in the number of inpatients, 6%.

3.6.2 Creating Demand for Family Planning to Improve Quality of Care: The Innovations in Family Planning Services Project

It was found that to execute a successful BCC strategy in the identified states, there was need for more and better-quality IEC materials and training, and also for their wider dissemination. Strengthening the capacity of service providers and programme implementers was at the heart of the IFPS strategy to improve the quality of messages and services to the people. Skills-building efforts were designed to increase knowledge and motivate service providers and frontline workers to enhance the community's ability to turn unmet needs into demand for accessible and affordable health services. The areas identified for skills building included approaches and methods for design, implementation, and evaluation of campaigns, using face-to-face meetings, and establishing mechanisms for institutionalizing this effort at the state level (Constella Futures 2006).

3.7 Integration of Family Planning Services with Other Health Services

The IPAS Development Foundation has developed strategies to improve post-abortion FP at public sector sites. Women having induced abortions or receiving post-abortion care are at high risk of subsequent unintended pregnancies, and intervals of less than six months between abortion and subsequent pregnancy may be associated with adverse outcomes. Ipas highlighted the prevalence of post-abortion contraceptive acceptance among women who received abortion care services at health facilities in six Indian states (Maharashtra, Madhya Pradesh, Uttarakhand, Rajasthan, Bihar, and Jharkhand). These efforts included: (*a*) provider capacity building for offering high-quality contraception and counselling; (*b*) continued engagement and support to the provider and facility team to ensure women-centred care; and (*c*) providing adequate counselling and information material.

Eighty-one per cent of the women accepted post-abortion contraceptive methods. Post-abortion contraceptive acceptance was highest among women who were aged 25 years and older, who received first-trimester services, attended primary-level health facilities, and had medical abortions. Comprehensive service delivery interventions, including ensuring availability of skilled providers and contraceptive commodities, offering clinical mentoring for providers, identifying and addressing provider bias, and improving providers' counselling skills, can increase post-abortion contraceptive acceptance and reduce unintended pregnancy.

3.8 Current Status of Implementation of Quality of Care Improvement Efforts: Perspectives from the Field

Two states—Rajasthan and Uttar Pradesh—were visited to ascertain the current status of implementation of various initiatives of the central government. The findings of these visits are described below.

3.8.1 Visit to Department of Health and Family Welfare, Government of Rajasthan (May 2016)

The PIP for financial year 2016–2017 of the state government of Rajasthan mentions an overall emphasis on QA and the Kayakalp initiative of the government to promote health-friendly initiatives. The programme budget includes meeting costs for QA meetings and FP review meetings, compensation for female sterilization, and cost of dissemination of manuals and guidelines. No separate budget is allocated for QA meetings and orientation. The cost of meetings is budgeted under general management costs. Budget is allocated for supporting counselling at district and subdistrict hospitals and mentoring for FP services.

Supplies: The management information system software is being upgraded to track contraceptives and FP commodities supply chain management. A logistics supply chain management system, e-Sadhan, is being built on the e-Aushadhi platform. This was proposed to be launched by July 2016.

Service delivery: Seasonal variations (a typical rise in sterilizations in the winter season [November, December, and January]) leads to increased workload, which is addressed by the empanelment of specialists. To address the high load of cases during sterilization camps and FP sessions, resources are budgeted for recruiting additional service providers. The budget makes a provision for compensation to acceptors of IUCD and sterilization services at quality fixed-day camps. A dedicated mobile team for sterilization services at the district level is provided. Sterilization camps are held at the CHC level (with requisite infrastructure and a functional operation theatre). However, before the Chhattisgarh incident (where 15 women died after undergoing sterilization operations), sterilization camps were held at PHC level as well.

To encourage follow-up visits by clients, certificates are issued only after the second and third month of the sterilization procedure. All checklists and consent forms related to sterilization and other FP methods are compiled in a booklet to simplify use and tracking of information.

Training: Capacity-building initiatives are undertaken to improve quality of services and client–provider interactions. This includes training by EngenderHealth on counselling services. Marie Stopes International conducted training in 12 high-priority districts on infection prevention and technical aspects. The Hindustan Latex Family Planning Promotion Trust (HLFPPT) has conducted and integrated training on QI in 120 PHCs. Training of ASHAs, anganwadi workers, and ANMs is being undertaken to improve client selection, counselling, and follow-up. Training provided to service providers includes RMNCH+A, FP counsellors, adolescent health counsellors, technical manuals, and counselling techniques. Medical officers are trained on NSV procedures, Minilap, and laparoscopic sterilization.

QA system: Discussions with key officials in the field suggest that regular meetings of the DQACs are not reported. Meetings are held primarily to assess failure cases of sterilization. The state government has advised all DQACs to report minutes of the meetings. Two QA meetings are held every six months with all service providers to take stock of infection control, drugs availability, and equipment. A division-level meeting is conducted once a year where private providers are invited. Previously, the state government had budgeted for quality certification and quality of services and functionality of public health facilities. Allocations were also made to recruit additional resources for QA cells. Three meetings for the review of QACs (Rs 20,000 per meeting) and three district review meetings per 10 districts (Rs 3000 per meeting) were conducted.

3.8.2 Visit to Department of Health and Family Welfare, Government of Uttar Pradesh (April 2016)

The Directorate of Health is focusing on strengthening FP quality in 40 focus districts. Technical assistance offered by development partners is focused on developing quality competency-based training to strengthen QoC in FP, and has focused on: (*a*) disseminating QA guidelines; (*b*) augmenting the technical capacity of service providers on clinical aspects of sterilization and IUCD; (*c*) orientation at facility level on rights framework; and (*d*) gender sensitivity, infection prevention, and QI at all levels.

Training: The department is supported by a technical support unit which provides technical assistance on key aspects of FP programming. As part of the technical support unit, EngenderHealth is providing technical support for conducting training of counsellors in 70 facilities (high client-load facilities) in 25 high-priority districts of Uttar Pradesh. Counselling training based on RMNCH+A guidelines is provided. Tools to support counselling sessions, which includes checklists, method-specific cue cards, and counselling kits are developed to assist the counsellors. Training of ASHAs and ANMs for coordination, follow-up, and outreach and field-level training of male counsellors and health education and information officers is proposed. A two-day training session on contraceptive technology (in the context of DMPA and POP) is proposed. These training programmes will be conducted with support from King George's Medical University, Lucknow.

Service delivery: Female sterilization and NSV services are provided on fixed days at health facilities in districts. Private centres and NGOs are being accredited for providing sterilization services. Performance incentives are also planned to be offered to service providers for PPIUCD insertion. Incentives and compensation are proposed for doctors at high-volume facilities in high-TFR (total fertility rate) districts to provide dedicated FP services. Additional counsellors are proposed for high case load facilities. Rebranding of facilities is being done to increase demand for services. Performance rewards are provided in the form of medals and memento certificates to high-performing service providers of LTT (Laparoscopy tubectomy), NSV, PPIUCD, and IUCD and to CMOs (Chief Medical Officers), medical officers, ASHAs, ANMs, and other facility staff like staff nurses who make extra efforts to provide quality services. Supportive supervision visits by PPIUCD trainers are organized.

The state government is also focusing on creating an enabling environment for improving uptake of FP services. Information, education, and communication material is being revised, and a 360-degree approach is being followed to develop attractive and relevant communication material. Further, LED boards are being installed in facilities to display health messages. The department is aiming to strengthen male involvement, especially in seven districts of Uttar Pradesh with high TFR, through the involvement and orientation of gram panchayats and VHSNCs.

Supplies: The Government of Odisha's RHCLMIS is approved for replication in Uttar Pradesh. A helpline is proposed that will follow up with clients and provide information over the phone.

Facility improvement: Under the Kayakalp initiative, the focus is on facility improvement, which is an important aspect of QoC. Social audits are proposed in the current PIP to understand the perspectives of clients on the quality of services provided. Fixed-day quality services (in the same facility) and fixed-day outreach services (at CHCs) are planned. Strengthening community linkages is proposed for encouraging greater ownership and improving the quality circle. Data (performance indicators) generated at block and district levels, however, is often not analysed.

Private sector role: A Health Partners Forum has been constituted at the state level to coordinate efforts around FP and to learn from each other. The state government has launched a new initiative called Hausla Sajhedari, under which private health care providers can get government accreditation. The programme works under the leadership, supervision, and monitoring of a state task force. It is an apex body constituted under the patronage of the principal secretary, Ministry of Health and Family Welfare, Government of Uttar Pradesh, and led by the executive director of the State Innovations in Family Planning Services Project Agency. A four member private sector provider cell serves as a secretariat to the state task force. The private sector provider cell looks after the web portal's day-to-day maintenance and the management of the Hausla Sajhedari initiative at the state level.

QA/QI systems: A quality circle intervention is delivered to improve and sustain the quality of strengthened sites. Quality circles are formed at each site with the medical officer in charge serving as chairperson. Members of quality circles represent all categories in the staff hierarchy. Each team member is assigned oversight responsibility for key aspects of quality (e.g., the management information system, water supply, electricity, maintenance, infection prevention practices, IEC, logistics, and cleanliness). The quality circle team meets every month to discuss issues and problems related to quality and possible solutions. The minutes of each meeting are noted along with solutions for identification of problems.

Orientation/review of ASHA/ANM/anganwadi workers (as applicable) is held on home delivery of contraceptives. Orientation workshops and QAC meetings are held to monitor progress in QoC as well as for review of sterilization failures. State-level half-yearly and divisional level quarterly review meetings are also held.

Quality assurance committees have been formed in all districts as well as at the state level. The process of staffing consultants for 600 vacancies is under way in the PIP for financial year 2016–2017. A budget (Rs 20,000 per month) for quarterly review meetings is assigned to assess quality across the spectrum of services.

Thus, officials at the state government level felt that comprehensive care would help provide quality FP services. There is also a need to conduct research on factors that enable uptake of a specific method over the other. Some efforts were reported for accreditation of private/NGO facilities to increase the provider base for FP services under the PPP initiative. The QACs in both states were being revised. However, most committees are understaffed and regular meetings of the committees are not reported.

3.9 Conclusion

Our review shows that MoHFW interventions to improve QoC include guidelines for facilities, service provision, and administrative matters, accreditation, and the QA system. These interventions have expanded method choices and enabled couples to have enhanced, informed choice through strengthened IEC and counselling. Development partners and NGOs have worked with the government to strengthen QA/QI systems, logistics, and training, and for improved service delivery, strengthened community relations, and integration of FP service with other health services in selected geographical areas.

Thus, most interventions by government as well as those led by and implemented in partnership with development partners and NGOs have been in the category of 'direct with possible immediate impact' (see Sect. 3.5). Almost all interventions have implemented one or more of the following: training (technical, communication), facility strengthening, augmenting staffing, improving supplies and provisioning necessary equipment; IEC/counselling; providing job aids; instituting standard operating procedures; and enhancing supportive supervision. There is some evidence that these have improved QoC.

Some interventions that focus on QA systems have been in the category of 'indirect with possible immediate impact' (Sect. 3.6). However, QI systems are rare. Both government and social franchisers accredit private providers using some QoC criteria. A few seek client feedback and some others have evaluated outcomes. However, community monitoring as an intervention to improve QoC is almost non-existent.

Thus, the interventions to improve QoC have, by and large, limited themselves to making a direct impact. Perhaps there is a need to look at QoC in broader frameworks so that these are seen as an integral part of the overall health system. Similarly, there is a need to empower women and communities to demand QoC when they receive FP services.

The FP programme is implemented by the states in India. Our site visits to two states—Rajasthan and Uttar Pradesh—show that the states have taken some actions for training, service delivery, facility improvements, supplies, and QA system. However, considerable challenges remain in the implementation of the QA system. These systems work in a limited way due to both budget constraints and staff vacancies in QACs at the district level. In most cases, their function seems to be limited to review of sterilization failure cases. However, these systems can be activated, as the Maharashtra example shows: the Government of Maharashtra implemented the QA system in a large number of districts with technical and financial assistance from UNFPA. The state governments need to prioritize improvement in the functioning of QA systems by providing needed budgets and monitoring their functioning at a high administrative level (Sect. 3.5.1).

References

Chauhan, K. (2015a). Repositioning family planning: Strengthening services within the primary health care centre in Karnataka by Karuna Trust. In J. Satia, K. Chauhan, A. Bhattacharya, & N. Mishra (Eds.), *Innovations in family planning: Case studies from India*. New Delhi: SAGE Publications.

Chauhan, K. (2015b). Reproductive Health Commodities Logistics Management Information System (RHCLMIS): Streamlining the supply chain for contraceptives in Odisha. In J. Satia, K. Chauhan, A. Bhattacharya, & N. Mishra (Eds.), *Innovations in family planning: Case studies from India* (pp. 67–78). New Delhi: SAGE Publications.

Constella Futures. (2006). *Ideas, insights, and innovations: Achievements and lessons learned from the Innovations in Family Planning Services (IFPS) project, 1992–2004*. New Delhi: Constella Futures.

EngenderHealth. (2003). *COPE® handbook: A process for improving quality in health services*. New York: EngenderHealth.

EngenderHealth. (2005). *EngenderHealth in India: Accomplishments under the Innovations in Family Planning Services project, 1996–2005*. New Delhi: EngenderHealth India Country Office.

Kumar, S., Sethi, R., Balasubramaniam, S., Charurat, E., Lalchandani, K., Semba, R., et al. (2014). Women's experience with postpartum intrauterine contraceptive device use in India. *Reproductive Health, 11*, 32. https://doi.org/10.1186/1742-4755-11-32.

Mishra, N., & Bishnoi, S. (2015). Ananya: An integrated approach to achieve health for all. In J. Satia, K. Chauhan, A. Bhattacharya, & N. Mishra (Eds.), *Innovations in family planning: Case studies from India* (pp. 5–21). New Delhi: SAGE Publications.

MoHFW (Ministry of Health and Family Welfare). (2012). *Indian public health standards: Guidelines for community health centres*. New Delhi: Directorate General of Health Services, Government of India.

MoHFW (Ministry of Health and Family Welfare). (2013). *Operational guidelines for quality assurance in public health facilities*. New Delhi: Government of India. http://www.rrcnes.gov.in/quality%20Assurance/Operational%20Guidelines%20on%20Quality%20Assurance%20(Print).pdf. Accessed January 21, 2018.

MoHFW (Ministry of Health and Family Welfare). (2015). *Quality standards for urban primary health centres*. New Delhi: Government of India.

MoHFW (Ministry of Health and Family Welfare). (2016a, March). *Manual for family planning indemnity scheme*. New Delhi: Government of India. http://nhm.gov.in/images/pdf/programmes/family-planing/schemes/FPIS_2nd_Edition_2016.pdf. Accessed January 21, 2018.

MoHFW (Ministry of Health and Family Welfare). (2016b). *National consultation on comprehensive abortion care for women*. New Delhi: Government of India.

MoHFW (Ministry of Health and Family Welfare). (2016c). *National family planning summit*. Press Information Bureau and MoHFW, Government of India. http://pib.nic.in/newsite/PrintRelease.aspx?relid=138580. Accessed January 24, 2018.

Nanda, P., Achyut, P., Mishra, A., & Calhoun, L. (2010). *Measurement, learning and evaluation of the Urban Health Initiative: Uttar Pradesh, India, baseline survey 2010 (TWP-3-2011)*. Chapel Hill, NC: Measurement, Learning & Evaluation Project.

Satia, J. (2015). Quality of care through quality assurance systems: The government of Maharashtra experience. In J. Satia, K. Chauhan, A. Bhattacharya, & N. Mishra (Eds.), *Innovations in family planning: Case studies from India* (pp. 51–66). New Delhi: SAGE Publications.

Satia, J., & Chauhan, K. (2015). Urban Health Initiative (UHI): A comprehensive intervention to address family planning needs of the urban poor in Uttar Pradesh. In J. Satia, K. Chauhan, A. Bhattacharya, & N. Mishra (Eds.), *Innovations in family planning: Case studies from India*. New Delhi: SAGE Publications.

Supreme Court of India. (2005). Record of proceedings. Order dated 1.3.2005, Writ Petition (Civil) No. 209/2003. *Ramakant Rai v. Union of India*. http://www.hrln.org/hrln/images/stories/pdf/ramakant-rai-order.pdf. Accessed January 24, 2018.

Chapter 4
Steps Taken by NGOs and the Private Sector to Improve Quality of Care

Abstract In this chapter, we discuss NGO-led interventions for demand creation/enhancing demand for quality of care, service delivery, and reaching young people. The private sector has two major operational modalities: social franchising and social marketing. Although many steps have been taken to improve quality of care through quality assurance in both these modalities, continuous QI is needed. We have hardly any information on quality of care in the private sector outside these two modalities.

Keywords Demand creation · Young people · Social marketing
Social franchising

4.1 Quality Improvement Interventions in NGO-Led Innovations

4.1.1 Respond: Project on Scaling up of Non-scalpel Vasectomy

Acceptance of vasectomy is very low in India, just about 1% of all modern methods of contraceptive use. Over the last decade, efforts have been made to increase providers for NSV. EngenderHealth, in collaboration with the state governments of Uttar Pradesh and Jharkhand and with financial support from the US Agency for International Development (USAID), implemented the "Respond" project during the period 2009–2013. It improved services through an updated curriculum; established centres of excellence and trained surgeons for NSV; improved supervision, QoC, and infection prevention; increased demand through improving the interpersonal communication skills of field-level workers (ASHAs); provided IEC materials and ensured ongoing coaching; and promoted a more favourable environment through improved policies including higher allocation of resources, recognition of performance, and inclusion in the agenda of district review meetings (Scott et al. 2011).

Nearly 17,000 clients were served by 231 surgeons trained in NSV over four years. An evaluation showed that nearly 60% of the facilities had all infrastructure, equipment, and supplies on the day of the team's visit. The quality of counselling improved significantly, and nearly 70% of the surgeons performed all essential NSV steps. Consequently, only one complication case was reported in four years. Nevertheless, human and financial resource shortages as well as the continuing need for reinforcement for QoC posed a challenge (Kumar 2016).

4.1.2 FHI 360: PROGRESS (Programme Research for Strengthening Services)

The PROGRESS project activities in India focused on four technical areas: PPFP, integration of FP with non-health sectors, expanding the contraceptive method mix, and capacity building and cross-cutting research utilization. These activities occurred primarily in the states of Uttar Pradesh and Jharkhand, but were also conducted at the national level (FHI360 2013).

A cross-sectional descriptive study was conducted to assess the quality of integration of FP into immunization services, and to develop recommendations for strengthening integrated service delivery among women in the extended postpartum period in the Indian state of Jharkhand. The findings indicated a number of service delivery challenges for integrated FP and child immunization services, ranging from postpartum women's fertility awareness to health systems issues. To address these challenges, the study recommended development of standard operating procedures to integrate services, incorporating the procedures and supportive materials into the regular government training for providers, and developing communication materials on integration.

4.1.3 Ujjwal Project

Futures Group and partners, HLFPPT, PHFI, the Johns Hopkins University Center for Communication Programs, and Oxford Policy Management implemented Project Ujjwal during 2011–2013. The project was directed towards expanding the market for FP and RH services and supplies by increasing use and service uptake among different income levels and age groups, and also towards complementing existing government schemes.

Towards this end, project strategies included expanding the choice of service delivery sites through a tiered franchisee network of 300 micro-enterprises (clinics/health facilities) and contracting in for fixed-day services at public health facilities by private outreach teams. Partnerships were established with premier institutions to introduce quality mechanisms (Federation of Obstetrics and Gynaecology Societies of India [FOGSI], PHFI, and state QACs) by investing in improvement of quality standards at clinics by introducing standard operating procedures and regular monitoring. To improve implementation, quality assessment studies (medical audits and client satisfaction surveys) were conducted; local capacities were strengthened for research and monitoring; and training of doctors and paramedics was undertaken, introducing and monitoring standard operating procedures at the provider level. The project developed a comprehensive management information system for tracking, monitoring, and consolidating routine data. The project developed the following tools for improving quality, which were adapted from the Government of India MOHFW guidelines on QA:

- QA monitoring formats: medical background and non-medical background (project/programme staff)
- QI plan development and monitoring of QI plans with individual clinics' providers based on medical audit results and need
- Checklists for external QA experts—this includes services and staff availability (including accreditation status), infrastructure, essential guidelines and protocols, infection prevention practices, equipment and supplies, and FP services (supplies, record review, and counselling)
- Clinic debriefing guidelines.

The overall strategies included innovative models (social franchising, social marketing, contracting in) that improved the quality of RMNCH+A care (FP/RH specifically, and now including maternal and child health) services in the private or public sector in India. The Ujjwal Project had a renewed focus on quality mechanisms in FP/RH service provision, with investments in collaboration with FOGSI national and state chapters to monitor the quality of service provision at private clinics and review training modules and audiovisual material on FP/RH for private providers. The project worked with the NHM in Odisha and Bihar on reviving state and district QACs and facilitating accreditation of private providers. The project was successful in establishing 288 franchisee clinics—maternal, neonatal, and child health (MNCH), FP, and safe abortion—conducting 955 fixed-day services at 120 public health facilities through outreach teams, demand generation for fixed-day services at public facilities, and accreditation of 51 clinics for government reimbursement. More than 900 doctors and paramedics were oriented on FP/RH, infection prevention practices, and standard operating procedures (OPM 2015).

4.1.4 Population Council: Systematic Screening to Integrate Reproductive Health Services in India

As a part of the Frontiers project, the Population Council conducted an operations research study that introduced systematic client service screening using a checklist. The systematic screening instrument helped register clients and identify unmet needs for RH, including FP, and provide services that clients need, making service provision comprehensive. Systematic screening produced a large increase in services per visit in experimental clinics at the same time that services per visit declined in the control clinics. The study also found that the systematic screening instrument produced smaller, but still non-trivial, increases at anganwadi centres. As an early outcome of the study, the city of Vadodara in the state of Gujarat decided to scale up systematic screening to other clinics. More broadly, the study demonstrated that systematic screening is an effective mechanism for integrating services at the provider level—the level that is most meaningful in reducing clients' unmet service needs. It was also found that almost all women with previously undetected service needs requested services, and that the clinics were able to provide almost all requested services in the same visit (USAID 2005). The results of this study are consistent with those of other studies conducted in Africa and Latin America.

4.1.5 The Dimpa Programme

Depo medroxyprogesterone acetate was introduced in India in 1994 after the Drug Controller of India cleared it for marketing by the private sector through prescriptions provided by qualified health practitioners as another option for women seeking FP. To generate demand for DMPA as a safe and effective contraceptive choice and increase its availability through partnership with commercial and social marketing agencies, USAID launched the Dimpa programme, implemented by Abt Associates, which sought to expand the choice of modern contraceptive methods by including the three-month injectable DMPA (Abt Associates 2007). The programme began in 2003 and has continued since then under diverse funding mechanisms. The objectives of the programme are to increase awareness of DMPA as a safe and effective method, create a network of private health care providers for providing high-quality options for a range of contraceptive methods, generate demand for DMPA as a safe and effective contraceptive choice, and increase availability of DMPA through partnership with commercial and social marketing agencies.

Since the time of its inception in 2003, the Dimpa programme has created a network of more than 1400 trained and motivated doctors in the private sector who impart quality care and counselling to interested contraceptive users, offering a wider choice of methods including DMPA. The outreach workers carry out door-to-door FP counselling, encouraging women to avail of the basket of choices.

A programme focus was to ensure that private doctors were trained in informed FP choice, screening for contraindications, and correct method usage. Quality assurance and follow-up ensured adherence to WHO criteria and guidelines for screening and counselling of clients, safe injection practices, and stocking of injectable contraceptives. Paramedical personnel and private doctors were trained on client registration, counselling, safe injection techniques, and follow-up care for potential and existing clients, and on dispelling myths about DMPA. Chemists were trained in stocking and dispensing DMPA (Sharma et al. 2013).

A Dimpa helpline was set up in 2008 to assist clients with questions on issues related to FP methods, including DMPA, and to refer clients to network clinics for method adoption and clinical services. The helpline, with six trained tele-counsellors, operates from 9.00 a.m. to 9.00 p.m. every day of the week.

4.1.6 Improving Quality of Care of Service Delivery for Intrauterine Contraceptive Devices

Several attempts have been made to improve IUCD service delivery, although its use to date remains limited. The Population Council promoted IUCD through improving QoC in Vadodara district in Gujarat (Visaria 1999). First, the criterion for measuring the performance of ANMs was changed to reflect the method mix. Then, ANMs and nurses were trained in insertion techniques through pictorial materials and IEC. A carry-on small diary was provided to them for counselling purposes. Knowledge of providers on the critical steps for providing IUD services increased significantly from 5 to 40%, and the proportion of women having poor knowledge (score of <7 out of 29) decreased significantly from 47 to 8%. Though the proportion believing in myths decreased significantly from the baseline, their prevalence was still high at the end line. The proportion of IUD users who reported the quality of IUD services received to be good (score of ≥ 25 out of 34) increased from 26 to 73%. A majority (92%) of providers used the IEC materials developed during the project when counselling clients, and 95% of them stated that their performance improved because of the IEC materials.

4.1.7 Odisha Urban Reproductive Health Project

The Parivar Seva Sansthan (PSS) implemented a state-wide contraceptive social marketing programme covering towns and rural areas in Odisha in 2003. The project provided a combination of services with an integrated approach to improving access and quality for poor and low-income women. It provided quality services through a combination of interventions using clinic-based and community-based approaches, as well as management of logistics and supply and promotional approaches, supported by elaborate monitoring and research. Two clinics in Bhubaneswar and Balasore cities provided clinical services on RH which set new standards for the quality of clinical services for both the public and the private sectors (PSS 2003).

4.2 Other Projects in the NGO Sector

4.2.1 Parivar Seva Sansthan

The PSS in its service programmes works for low- and middle-income groups mainly living in urban slums, peri-urban and rural areas, who are unable to afford commercial services and products and also do not wish to avail of free-of-cost services from the public sector. Annually, through its birth prevention programmes, PSS provides over a million couples years of protection. The PSS established RH clinics with a focus on safe and legal abortion and FP in each of 10 districts in Bihar, Rajasthan, Madhya Pradesh, and Uttar Pradesh. It developed medical protocols for each service, and monitoring and audit systems including quality audits. The key focus of the intervention was on increasing utilization of cost-effective, quality RH services. The project approach included community mobilization and motivation, strengthening FP supply, and referrals to separate static clinics for men and women. These services were complemented by a state-wide contraceptive social marketing programme to promote and make quality products widely accessible on a sustainable basis and at affordable prices, using commercial and other channels to focus on prevention of unwanted births. Today, PSS has 36 clinics located across 11 states of India, delivering a range of quality and affordable RH services with emphasis on FP (both terminal and spacing methods), antenatal–postnatal care, safe abortion services, and treatment of sexually transmitted infections and HIV/AIDS. Clinical services are provided to over 200,000 clients annually through these clinics, besides reaching lakhs of men and women with health, and particularly RH, BCC.

4.2.2 Marie Stopes India

Marie Stopes International has two country programmes in India: Population Health Services India, which was established in 1999, and Marie Stopes India (MSI), which opened in 2008. Since opening, Population Health Services India has expanded its operations and offers SRH care in centres in 14 locations across four states. Population Health Services India offers a range of quality SRH services through its centres. It leads the field in clinical quality standards and client focus, and its units double as knowledge and training centres for the MoHFW.

Marie Stopes International works with the 24 district health authorities in these states to deliver FP, and offers the third largest social marketing programme in the country. It works in partnership with government ministries to improve service provision. Its service delivery and capacity building and social franchising efforts focus on public sector and select private providers through training and QI support, and advocacy to foster an enabling environment.

4.2 Other Projects in the NGO Sector

Marie Stopes India is working to improve the quality of services, spearheading national SRH policies and training local providers to strengthen the services they deliver to clients. Working with the Government of Rajasthan, MSI is increasing the provision of long-acting and permanent FP methods in 13 districts. In Madhya Pradesh, MSI works to ensure that marginalized and young women are given the choice of a range of quality FP services. It uses clinical outreach in underserved areas to support and improve government FP service delivery. Teams travel to hard-to-reach parts of the country, offering services to those who need them most.

Through its social marketing programme, MSI expands access to services such as short-term and long-term methods of contraception. It uses clinical outreach in underserved areas to support and improve government FP service delivery. In India, MSI is working with the state governments of Rajasthan, Uttar Pradesh, and Bihar. Fixed-day services are conducted by clinical outreach teams, where the mobile outreach teams deliver counselling and high-quality voluntary FP services to women and men who would not otherwise be able to access them. Highly experienced and qualified clinical teams provide access to long-term and permanent methods of FP that would otherwise not be available in these areas. A subset of the clinical outreach teams (the mini clinical outreach team) moves to health sub-centres around the facilities where the clinical outreach team is offering services, to bring spacing methods, including IUCD services, closer to women, particularly young newlywed women. For people in urban slum areas (in-reach centres), MSI provides comprehensive FP counselling and FP clinical services that include providing condoms, OCPs, emergency contraceptives, injections, IUDs, tubal ligations, and vasectomy.

Marie Stopes India works closely with district health functionaries to develop an outreach schedule at the beginning of each month. This camp schedules are then publicized to the clients through demand generation activities. The interpersonal communicators of MSI work closely with ASHAs, who work for the public sector, to prime potential clients about various FP methods and about the services provided by clinical outreach teams and mini clinical outreach teams through door-to-door visits; they also communicate the outreach camp locations and timings.

4.2.3 Action Research and Training for Health

High unmet need for limiting contraception persists in most states of India despite wide access to sterilization. Action Research and Training for Health (ARTH) implemented an intervention to introduce Copper-T 380A—a contraceptive with an effective life span of 10 years—as an alternative to female sterilization in a rural area of the state of Rajasthan, in a clinic linked to an outreach programme. The intervention addressed women's apprehensions, ensured service standards, and guaranteed women's right to have the Copper-T removed at will. Data on 216 insertions over 34 months revealed a preference for the Copper-T 380A among older women and women who had achieved the desired family size, especially among tribal women. More than a quarter of the 30 removals in that period were for non-medical reasons, such as family opposition, child death, or remarriage. As a long-term but reversible option, the Copper-T 380A allows women room to change their minds in relation to future childbearing until they have reached menopause. Including this option in FP services can help to meet a portion of the unmet need for contraception among women not willing to choose sterilization, while reducing dependence on doctors and expensive equipment. The intervention addressed women's apprehensions, ensured service standards, and guaranteed women's right to have the Copper-T removed at will. The intervention also underscores the importance of addressing women's apprehensions about IUDs. Despite their traditional outlook, rural and, even more so, tribal communities tend to take decisions based on empirical evidence and what they perceive as being effective. The ARTH intervention therefore paid attention to the quality of counselling, screening, asepsis, and follow-up procedures for introducing the Copper-T. Even after factoring women's concerns into a carefully designed, interactive communication package, it took several months for trust in the method to translate into actual acceptance in the community (Iyengar and Sharad 2000).

4.2.4 Population Services International

User satisfaction is an important contributor to greater compliance and longer continuation of contraceptive methods. Population Services International (PSI) India conducted a study titled "Role of Helpline Outbound Calling in Reduction of Dissatisfaction and Discontinuation Rate among IUD Clients". The baseline data indicated that the following knowledge/beliefs are significant determinants of IUD use: awareness that the IUD is as effective as sterilization; and awareness that IUD side effects subside within three to four months. The baseline also found that most IUD discontinuation occurs within three months of insertion. These findings alerted PSI India to the need for an "after-service" follow-up call apart from the routine follow-up visit by the client to the provider. The call is intended to dispel myths about side effects, check client satisfaction, and to evaluate the quality of IUD services. Making a follow-up call after client service is important for a number of reasons, including improving the organization's/clinic's credibility. The follow-up adds value to the service or product the client has received and gives an opportunity to build a stronger relationship with each client. This could result in referrals to more potential clients.

In another effort, the Women's Health Initiative (Pehel), PSI India designed a telephone helpline service to provide correct information and post-service follow-up, and to refer women to service delivery sites and report complications (see Sect. 4.2.9). The technology used in this initiative includes phones, computers, apps/software, and PDAs/tablets.

4.2.5 Public Health Foundation of India, United Nations Population Fund, and Federation of Obstetric and Gynaecological Societies of India

A certificate course on contraception in clinical practice to train primary care physicians in evidence-based contraceptive practices across India was launched by PHFI, FOGSI, and UNFPA. The main objective of this programme is to enhance the knowledge, skills, and core competencies of primary care physicians on evidence-based contraceptive methods and practice, and also to establish a network of primary care physicians with reputed faculty, creating a platform for their knowledge upgradation. The course was launched at the national level on 25 August 2013. In the first phase of the programme, 660 candidates enrolled for the certificate course. The course has been implemented in 36 designated centres covering 18 states. A didactic course curriculum was prepared and reviewed by eight FOGSI national experts who played a vital role in the nomination and training of trainers. The course content consisted of four specific modules, including CDs/videos/case studies along with toolkits for practical sessions, which proved to be very useful for better understanding of the subject. The training programme (consisting of four sessions) was conducted by 72 experienced FOGSI faculty (two faculty assigned per centre) over four months from August till December 2013. The final assessment of all pre- and post-test questionnaires suggests that participants' knowledge was enhanced after taking this course and showed overall improvement.

4.2.6 Addressing the Needs of Young People: Empowerment Through Life Skills Education and Counselling

Two distinctive experiences that aimed at meeting the contraceptive needs of young people are presented here. Drishti is a life skills programme aimed at building the capacity of teachers, including District Institute of Education and Training lecturers, to impart life skills education in government schools in the state of Rajasthan. The overall aim of this programme was to empower schoolgoing young adolescents (12–14 years) to make informed choices about their health and behaviour through classroom sessions on life skills education conducted by trained teachers. In addition, outreach efforts were made to engage with parents and the community through the students and impact the quality of their decision making. Advocacy with the administrative and education department at the state level resulted in the inclusion of life skills in the pre-service curriculum for teacher training. Training of teachers has been an integral part of the training calendar of the District Institute of Education and Training in the three intervention districts, and subsequently of the State Institute of Education and Training. In addition, outreach efforts were made to engage with parents and the community through the students, to impact the quality of their decisions with respect to young people. A questionnaire was administered to the teachers after every training to measure participation levels, the quality of study materials, and for feedback on improvement in the programme design.

The Healthy Timing and Spacing of Pregnancy (HTSP) project implemented by the Population Council was designed to understand cultural and reproductive constructs that are conducive to early first birth and short-spaced pregnancies. The project developed a comprehensive model to test its effectiveness in educating young couples, elderly family members, and community members about birth spacing and its advantages. The messages were designed for: (*a*) husbands with an emphasis on economic implications; (*b*) wives, on economic and health implications; and (*c*) parents (the mother-in-law) on the health of the child and economic implications. It also involved changing the style of working of anganwadi workers through a specially designed notebook and communication products. The key intervention was an educational campaign on HTSP for pregnant women during antenatal care visits to the clinics and community worker visits to the home. In addition, husbands, mothers-in-law, and community opinion leaders were also educated.

As a result of this effort, 30% of the women had read HTSP messages painted on the walls of the anganwadi centre or other prominent places. Forty-five per cent of the women had seen at least one of the messages on birth spacing disseminated through posters and wall paintings. Around 88% of the women who received the HTSP booklet shared it with their husbands, but only 49% shared it with their mother-in-law. The high use of contraception at 9–10 months postpartum (68%) in the experimental area shows that couples who are provided with the correct information and contraceptive services will adopt the lactational amenorrhea method (LAM), and then transition from LAM to modern contraceptive methods (Bishnoi 2015).

4.2.7 mHealth for Content Distribution

An mHealth platform was implemented in several countries, including in India in the state of Bihar, to create and publish a wide range of content for community engagement, training of community health workers, and education (Ashcroft 2016). The aim of this app was to assist frontline health workers (FHWs) and clients in deciding on FP methods during counselling sessions, and to accelerate the rate of adoption of spacing methods among young married couples. It will expand to address the entire range of services in the RMNCH+A continuum.

The ASHAs can download the content on their smartphones for dialogue with and counselling of clients. Among other content, it includes four types of videos:

doctor or expert films, role model films, enter-educate, and TV-style public service announcements (PSAs). The pilot effort in a block showed that there was a perceivable increase in the uptake of FP services, and ASHAs were able to address client queries more efficiently. The credibility of counselling sessions increased, and there was active interest in and sharing of informational content in the community.

The platform allows an open, collaborative model for distribution of content and allows for government oversight and ownership, thereby permitting low-cost scalability.

4.2.8 Empowering Clients to Demand Quality of Care for Maternal Health Using Mobile Technology: A Pilot Study in Jharkhand

This pilot introduced a mobile monitor for QoC using basic mobile phones for an interactive voice platform by which women could provide feedback on services received, and thereby become actively engaged advocates for positive improvement of quality services (Ominde 2016). It also informed expecting mothers of existing health entitlements. It used QoC indicators arrived at by a consensus-building process—timeliness, service guarantee, respectful care, and cleanliness of the facility—measured by a set of 18 indicators. A well-advertised toll-free number was provided, on which women could call and provide their ratings on the QoC they received. This feedback was converted into rating scores and shared with public and private facilities to help them improve care, as well as with households to help them decide where to seek care. Also, women's knowledge about their entitlements improved significantly. Thus, this pilot shows the feasibility and utility of a client feedback system. It can be adapted for FP as well as scaled up.

4.2.9 Pehel: Addressing Women's Health in Rajasthan, Delhi, and Uttar Pradesh

Pehel is an initiative of PSI India to empower women in the reproductive age group to make informed choices for addressing their needs of FP and safe abortion in 19 districts of Uttar Pradesh, Rajasthan, and Delhi. The partnership aims to reduce maternal mortality and morbidity by increasing demand for and access to temporary and long-acting FP methods. The Pehel project was launched in July 2008 and initially implemented in 10 states across the country, providing free services for IUD insertion. Based on the learning from phase I, the strategy was to concentrate project activities to 19 districts across three states, Rajasthan, Delhi, and Uttar Pradesh. In the scale-up phase of Pehel II, efforts were continued to create an enabling environment for increasing access and improving QoC for IUD and safe medical abortions through safe abort kits in the private sector. In 2013, Pehel III was launched as a part of a 14-country initiative by PSI to provide informed choice and enhance quality in postpartum FP and post-abortion FP through private sector engagement in Rajasthan, Uttar Pradesh, and Delhi. It targets 30 districts of Delhi, Uttar Pradesh, and Rajasthan to promote the use of long-term reversible contraceptives (IUCD) and safe medical abortions to help reduce the maternal mortality rate.

Pehel seeks to harness the potential of the private sector by providing capacity enhancement opportunities for IUCD and creating a service delivery network, namely, Saadhan clinics, to improve access to high-quality IUCD services, assuring people of quality and affordability. Population Services International partnered with FOGSI to develop a social franchise network of clinics called "Saadhan" (which means "aid" in Hindi) to ensure the availability of quality IUCD services to communities, specifically the lower-income population group. This was based on background research to offer services that would be associated with quality and reliability. The Federation of Obstetrics and Gynaecology Societies of India has a large network of doctors (obstetricians and gynaecologists), which is exposed to knowledge, skills, and QoC issues through periodic orientation sessions. Regular meetings are used to share the latest scientific updates on FP methods and provide refresher training to enhance the skills of doctors in promoting long-term birth spacing methods, such as IUCDs. The district-level team of FOGSI members is involved in promoting quality IUCD services in Pehel implementation areas, and in updating other private service providers on evidence-based technical knowledge and skills. This has helped in developing a network of service providers for providing quality, long-term birth spacing methods. The Saadhan network members provide health services to urban and peri-urban women. Interpersonal communicators work to mobilize the community, and make house-to-house visits in the target area to provide IUCD counselling and referrals to network doctors. The partnership of PSI with FOGSI has enhanced the visibility of Pehel, encouraging doctors to join the network and increase the standards of quality related to IUCD. The network is supported by a tele-helpline. A computer software package, designed to complement helpline services, contains a data bank with a list of possible questions and appropriate responses, as well as a contact list of health service providers for referral. The software tracks clients so that counsellors can follow up with repeat callers, and provides a list of words that enables counsellors to access slang and vernacular terminology that clients may use during their tele-conversation session.

Thus, PSI's strategy for increasing the provider base for IUCD by strengthening the capacity of existing private sector providers to enhance access and improve quality is as follows. This was based on background research to offer services that would be associated with quality and reliability. The Federation of Obstetrics and Gynaecology Societies of India has a large network of doctors (obstetricians and gynaecologists), which is exposed to knowledge, skills, and QoC issues through periodic orientation sessions. Regular meetings are held to share the latest scientific updates on FP methods and provide refresher training to enhance the skills of doctors in promoting long-term birth spacing methods, such as IUCDs. The district-level team of FOGSI members is involved in promoting quality IUCD services in Pehel implementation areas, and in updating other private service providers on evidence-based technical knowledge and skills. This has helped in developing a network of service providers for providing quality, long-term birth spacing methods.

In order to ensure quality control, the network coordinators visit network providers twice a month for reviewing product attributes, placement of product, and to capture the monthly IUCD inventory status of each provider in order to monitor uptake of IUCDs. These coordinators are trained by the medical services team of PSI on the technical aspects of all modern contraceptive methods. The medical services team and network coordinators visit the provider facilities to assess them on minimum quality standards. A provider needs to meet the minimum quality standards to be a part of the network. The medical team visits the providers regularly and provides supportive supervision and handholding to ensure that all quality parameters are met during IUCD insertions. Repeated visits are made by the medical team till quality service to clients is ensured. The following actions were taken to improve QoC:

1. Technical competence: training, procedure to be performed by licensed health providers, and a letter of association identifying responsibilities of both parties;
2. Client safety: screening, compliance with facility standards, infection prevention, management of complications and adverse events;
3. Informed choice: access to a range of contraceptives, counselling;
4. Privacy and confidentiality;
5. Continuity of care: information on follow-up and referral through helpline and communications team, ensuring client satisfaction.

The demand was generated by the use of mass media, holding group meetings, and interpersonal communication. Providers were recognized for good performance. The programme built capacity, improved QoC, and increased availability, covering a network of 1123 providers. Pehel also worked with national and state governments to develop guidelines and quality protocols.

4.2.10 Family Planning Association of India SETU Core+ Project

The SETU Core+ project aimed to increase contraceptive coverage, improve awareness of FP among all men, women, and young people, and strengthen systems for the Family Planning Association of India to ensure efficient forecasting and logistics management of commodities across the association. An outreach intervention was implemented in 17 blocks across India in 2014. Each block had a satellite clinic and an outreach team. The satellite clinic had a doctor, staff nurse, counsellor, lab technician, ANM, and helper. The outreach team comprised a community-based distributor (CBD), link worker, and project coordinator. The CBD was the commodity provider at the grassroots level, and the rest of the team was for supportive supervision. A block, with population varying from 1 to 2 lakh, had about 120–200 CBDs. Strategies adopted included community mobilization through CBDs for demand generation and referrals to satellite clinics, mobile medical vans twice a week, special service sessions in the community, and partnerships with private medical practitioners in the area. During the year 2013, CBDs provided 979,495 (64%) of the services, while satellite clinics provided 634,425 (42%) services. The SETU project contributed significantly (46%) to the overall branch performance. The SETU project model proved to be cost-effective for provision of contraceptive services. The cost per contraceptive service provided by CBDs and satellite clinics was found to be $0.48 and $0.47, respectively. Thus, a multi-level service delivery point is an efficient and cost-effective method of providing FP and contraceptive information and services.

4.2.11 DKT India

In partnership with private medical practitioners (AYUSH), DKT India uses a network of responsive sales representatives to distribute condoms and other FP products in districts throughout India using dynamic social marketing. AYUSH doctors will continue the provision of contraceptive and SRH services to the community, and provide client referral to FPAI clinics for those requiring sterilization, abortion, and other high-skilled services.

4.3 Approaches to Assuring Quality of Care in Social Franchising Operations

Social franchising is a way of contracting private providers to join a branded franchised chain, and is being taken up in many developing countries, leading to improvements in service quality, usage rates, and client perceptions. A franchiser is the owner and originator of the particular brand and its policies. The role of the franchiser is recruitment, selection, training, supply, continuous support, and monitoring of providers in the franchisee network, including the advertisement of the brand. Moreover, the franchiser should strive to create better access to quality products and services for clients, develop standards and procedures for the programmes, provide technical assistance and programming of new technologies to maximize coverage, and ensure that care reaches all population groups, particularly those with limited access. Franchisee clinics deliver quality services, ensuring informed choices for clients from a wide range of methods, and creating awareness in the communities for accessing the services.

4.3.1 Social Franchising Programmes in India

Social franchising presents itself as a key organizing force in the private health care sector in developing countries. Several large social franchising programmes operate in India in FP, including HLFPPT, Marie Stopes International, PSI, DKT, and Abt Associates.

Janani Health Network: Janani started a social marketing and social franchise programme that uses India's large private health sector network of practitioners and facilities to provide safe and low-cost options for FP, health, and RH services in rural areas. The focus is on providing clinical FP methods and CAC through its Surya Clinics. They provide express service delivery for referral clients that have come in through the outreach networks. They also maintain regular supplies of contraceptives to both rural and urban pharmacies and shops.

Merry Gold Health Network: The Merry Gold Health Network established by HLFPPT aims at creating access to low-cost, good-quality maternal and child health services by networking with private health service providers as franchisees. The Merry Gold Health Network was conceived to harness the potential of social franchising to establish a range of private providers in Uttar Pradesh and Rajasthan that would address the RH/FP needs of low-income groups among the urban poor and in rural areas. The aim was to create a social enterprise. The franchise targets the low-income population, migrants/refugees, women and children in providing its services. Services include infertility treatment, HIV voluntary counselling and testing, contraceptives, and safe delivery services amongst many others. Emphasis is on affordable pricing, QA, customer servicing, and efficient service delivery through standardized operating protocols. An information technology enabled hospital management information system (HMIS) is also being established with an emphasis on FP services.

4.3.2 Ensuring Quality of Care in Social Franchising Operations

Within social franchising programmes, managers use a rich and varied set of approaches to assure that clinical and patient care is delivered in accordance with international guidelines, including practicum trainings, on-the-job observation and feedback, and performance-based incentives. Broadly, these measures include the following:

- Management contracts
- Medical audits
- QA mechanisms
  - Regular site visits
  - Periodic clinical audits (internal and external)
  - Mystery clients, client exit interviews
  - Client and provider focus groups
  - Provider surveys and self-assessments
  - Community-level interviews.

4.3.3 Devising a Quality Metric for Social Franchisee Operations in Family Planning Globally

The increasing engagement of the commercial sector in providing FP through private clinics is particularly noticeable in the burgeoning of social franchising. Recent reviews (Madhavan and Bishai 2010; Mwaikambo et al. 2011; Stephenson et al. 2004) find strong evidence that franchising increases access to and use of FP services with moderate evidence of improved quality and moderate evidence of increased use by the poor.

The importance of measuring QoC emerges as many countries move towards purchasing services from the private sector. If quality can be measured objectively, and if quality scores can be made publicly available, there are enormous advantages. Institutional purchasers will choose the best providers and reward them through differential tariffs. Individuals will follow, whether paying out of pocket or leveraging their insurance. Providers who fail to reach acceptable standards will fall by the wayside, and markets will promote continued improvements. Development of common metrics in social franchising can inform the wider health sector.

A survey showed that all social franchises have quality and QI activities at the heart of their operations. Typically, the QA system

- Sets FP norms and standards for all affiliated programmes
- Aligns international NGO standards with domestic policies; sets monitoring, compliance, and provider engagement policies
- Determines use of personnel for monitoring, compliance, and provider engagement
- Engages with providers for assessment and mentoring purposes
- Engages with clients to facilitate use of FP services and follow-up care
- Participates in orientation and refresher trainings; agrees to upgrade equipment or facilities if needed; agrees to follow business and clinical protocols; reports adverse events
- Reports satisfaction or complaints with community mobilizers or through helplines.

4.3 Approaches to Assuring Quality of Care in Social Franchising Operations

Although these systems are comprehensive, predictable, and well structured and have trackable data, they may not provide comparable data across providers: routine monitoring is difficult and can be expensive; assessment checklists can be bulky; and considerable QA personnel may be required. Observation of services in selected facilities showed that critical areas for lack of adherence were infection prevention, clinical procedures, and patient–provider interactions.

In 2014, the Social Franchising Metrics Working Group was set up—a group of academics, programme managers, and donors committed to identifying and testing robust metrics for assessment of franchise operations. The adoption of standard metrics will be important for programme managers to make effective comparisons of facilities on common performance metrics for iterative QI. To date, the process used is to seek inputs from selected social franchisee programmes as well as convene an expert working group (Viswanathan and Seefeld 2015).

The adoption of structural quality metrics of provider and facility readiness will help programmes become more efficient and effective, leading to improved infrastructure and supply chains, which will ultimately provide clients with access to higher-quality FP services. However, provider and facility readiness alone are not sufficient to capture service quality. Process quality, which encompasses the provider–client interaction as well as the skills executed by the provider, must also be considered. Process quality is necessary for improving FP counselling, clinical practice, and patient satisfaction.

The Social Franchising Metrics Working Group is now directing its focus towards measuring quality more holistically across three domains: readiness, process, and outcome. An expert group has proposed a minimal set of indicators to be tested, as follows:

- Readiness: choice, commodities, equipment, service provider
- Process: interpersonal skills, information provided, and technical competence
- Outcome: method information index, 12-month post-services.

In October 2015, the Rockefeller Conference Center organized a meeting on QoC in FP which brought together FP providers, academics, global policy leaders, researchers, and donor agencies to agree on how to advance towards a common measure of the quality of FP service provision. The meeting also discussed the evolving landscape of FP, and the need for a standardized metric (Leisher et al. 2016).

4.4 Social Marketing

As mentioned earlier, DKT India uses a network of responsive sales representatives to distribute condoms and other FP products in districts across the country using dynamic social marketing methods. DKT looks after the quality indicators of departments and the monitoring of the indicators on a monthly basis. Compliance of medical records is checked by regular audits. Staff is trained for quality-related teachings, compliances, hospital policies, protocols, and usages as required by QI guidelines.

4.5 Advocating Reproductive Choices: Catalysing Stakeholder Engagement for Repositioning Family Planning

Although it is difficult to directly attribute outcomes to various advocacy efforts, there is now widespread awareness and appreciation of the need to expand contraceptive choice and improve QoC. The advocacy efforts have also accelerated initiatives by the government to emphasize spacing methods; expand choice through promoting NSV and IUDs; improve QoC; and focus on adolescents.

The objective of the Advocating Reproductive Choices initiative was "to expand the contraceptive choices for the Indian population by widely promoting and making available safe, effective and quality contraceptives in the public and private health service delivery system at affordable costs".

The task force reviewed available material on QoC and recommended some changes. In 2013 it prepared a checklist for QA, which was pre-tested. The state government of Uttar Pradesh expressed its interest in this checklist and initiated a pilot test in Lucknow city. It now proposes to expand use of the checklist to 10 cities in Uttar Pradesh.

There is a need to create a set of indicators related to QA that can serve as benchmarks against which QoC is monitored. In addition, there is a need to put in place standard protocols for service delivery. Community ownership and community-based mechanisms to monitor QoC on an ongoing basis are critical to ensuring quality services.

Advance Family Planning is an initiative that aims to increase the financial investment and political commitment needed to ensure access to high-quality, voluntary FP through evidence-based advocacy.

Thus, while progress is visible, much more remains to be done to achieve the ultimate goal of ensuring that every person can exercise informed choice, have access to a wide range of methods, and receive high QoC to meet their needs for contraception.

4.6 Conclusion and the Way Forward

Non-governmental organizations have implemented a variety of pilot projects that have demonstrated: (*a*) ways to improve provider competence for NSV; (*b*) challenges in integrating FP with immunization services during the postpartum period;

4.6 Conclusion and the Way Forward

(c) systematic screening to integrate provision of RH services; (d) introduction of DMPA in provision; and (e) service delivery of IUCD with requisite QoC. Provision of contraceptive information and services to young people is sought to be improved: (a) through life skills education; and (b) through comprehensive communication efforts to educate young people as well as family and community members on the benefits of birth spacing. Pilot projects to use mHealth tools to increase provider competencies for communication as well as to demand QoC in maternal health services have proved their utility in aiding QoC improvement efforts. The use of mHealth tools to aid QoC improvement efforts need to be innovated and scaled up.

Almost all of the above projects have included measures to ensure QoC. Non-governmental organizations have also individually and collectively advocated for the repositioning of FP.

Private sector delivery of FP services has included social franchising, social marketing, and contracting in. Social franchising networks as a part of global networks have embarked on collective efforts to improve QoC in their services. Their instruments to ensure/improve QoC have included selection of franchisees, management contracts, medical audits, and QA mechanisms. However, measuring QoC efficiently and effectively has proved challenging. The quality of products provided through social marketing is presumably assured by the manufacturers. However, it is not clear how the provision of correct information to clients is ensured through the delivery channels used.

While reviewing interventions to improve QoC undertaken by the government and with support from development partners and NGOs in Chap. 3, it was found that most efforts were geared towards influencing variables that had a direct, immediate influence on QoC. We had also mentioned that QA systems as well as monitoring and evaluation of outcomes having an indirect immediate influence on QoC needed to be strengthened. However, the pilot projects by NGOs have used these mechanisms more frequently.

Very few interventions influence proximate variables to improve QoC. Directly influencing proximate variables include targets/work expectations, and incentives/disincentives. The policies relating to these are well established in government. Interventions to influence health system functioning having indirect proximate effect on QoC for FP have generally not received attention except for facility strengthening and health services staffing. The responsiveness of health institutions to patient needs as well as the voice and participation of clients in the functioning of health services also have an indirect proximate effect on QoC in FP. However, it is not clear how these have been influenced by the interventions studied. There are a few interventions that have sought to integrate FP into maternal and child health or other RH services such as HIV or post-abortion care. However, it is not clear whether such integration has improved QoC for FP.

Hardly any interventions influence distal variables to improve QoC. Distal influences such as the agency/autonomy of women and community norms as well as the overall organizational, social, and political context of health system functioning seem to have not been considered as having a distal effect on improving QoC for FP.

Besides strengthening the QA system mentioned in Chap. 3, the above review shows that there are at least two challenges in improving QoC going forward:

- *Measurement challenge*: While it is relatively easier to measure structural variables of provider and facility readiness, QoC during the process of service delivery is difficult to measure and requires more resources. There is a need to innovate ways to measure process and outcome variables of QoC efficiently, possibly using mHealth tools.
- *Health system challenge*: It can be argued whether QoC in FP can be improved and sustained without similar efforts to improve QoC in other health programmes or for health system as a whole. Clearly, isolated efforts will have suboptimal results. However, while there are some efforts to improve QoC in RMNCH+A or a few other health programmes, there is no overarching movement to improve QoC in health services provision in India as a whole.

References

Abt Associates. (2007). *Using partnerships to expand the use of injectable contraceptives: The Dimpa network*. http://www.abtassoc.net/presentations/DimpaNetworkASinha.pdf. Accessed on December 7, 2017.

Ashcroft, C. N. (2016). The linkages between fertility awareness and family planning uptake: Program findings of scaling mHealth services in India. Presentation made at the *International Conference on Family Planning, Panel 99*.

Bishnoi, S. (2015). Addressing needs of young people: Empowerment through life skills education and counselling. In J. Satia, K. Chauhan, A. Bhattacharya, & N. Mishra (Eds.), *Innovations in family planning: Case studies from India* (pp. 221–239). New Delhi: SAGE Publications.

FHI360. (2013). *Improving access to family planning: End of project meeting*. https://www.fhi360.org/sites/default/files/media/documents/fhi360-global-approach-family-planning-finger.pdf. Accessed on December 7, 2017.

Iyengar, K., & Sharad, D. I. (2000). The Copper-T 380A IUD: A ten-year alternative to female sterilisation in India. *Reproductive Health Matters, 8*(16), 125–133. https://doi.org/10.1016/S0968-8080(00)90194-0.

Kumar, D. (2016). Capacity building in no-scalpel vasectomy leads to greater contraceptive choice in Uttar Pradesh and Jharkhand, India. In *International Conference on Family Planning, Panel 1536*.

Leisher, S. H., Sprockett, A., Longfield, K., & Montagu, D. (Eds.). (2016, October). *Quality measurement in family planning: Past, present, future*. Papers from the Bellagio Meeting on Family Planning Quality. Metrics for Management, Oakland, CA.

Madhavan, S., & Bishai, D. (2010). *Private sector engagement in sexual and reproductive health and maternal and neonatal health a review of the evidence*. Baltimore: Department of Population, Family, and Reproductive Health, Johns Hopkins Bloomberg School of Public Health.

References

Methur D, Pandya B. (2016). Role of helpline outbound calling in reduction of dissatisfaction and discontinuation rate among IUD clients. Plesented at the International Conference on Family Planning (ICFP). http://www.psi.org/icfp-2016/ Accessed on 7 July 2017.

Mwaikambo, L., Speizer, I. S., Schurmann, A., Morgan, G., & Fikree, F. (2011). What works in family planning interventions: A systematic review. *Studies in Family Planning, 42*(2), 67–82.

Ominde, A. (2016). A matter of rights, choice, and quality: Effective quality of care interventions in family planning programs. In *International Conference on Family Planning, Panel 199*.

OPM (Oxford Policy Management). (2015). *Impact evaluation of project Ujjwal*. http://www.opml.co.uk/sites/default/files/Impact_Evaluation_of_Project_Ujjwal.pdf. Accessed on December 7, 2017

PSS (2003). *Report of Odisha urban reproductive health project*. Parivar Seva Sansthan

Scott, B., Alam, D., & Raman, S. (2011). Factors affecting acceptance of vasectomy in Uttar Pradesh: Insights from community-based, participatory qualitative research. *The RESPOND Project Study Series, Contributions to global knowledge—Report no. 3*. New York: EngenderHealth/The RESPOND Project.

Sharma, V., Sagar, M., & Singh, A. (2013). *Evaluation of Dimpa injectable contraceptive network in India. Strengthening Health Outcomes through the Private Sector (SHOPS)*. USA: Abt Associates.

Stephenson, R., Tsui, A. O., Sulzbach, S., Bardsley, P., Bekele, G., Giday, T., et al. (2004). Franchising reproductive health services. *Health Services Research, 39*(6, part 2), 2053–2080.

USAID (United States Agency for International Development). (2005). *Systematic screening to integrate reproductive health services in India*.

Visaria, L. (1999). The quality of reproductive health care in Gujarat: Perspectives of female health workers and their clients. In M. A. Koenig & M. E. Khan (Eds.), *Improving quality of care in India's family welfare programme* (pp. 143–168). New York: Population Council.

Viswanathan, R., & Seefeld, C. A. (2015). *Clinical social franchising compendium. An annual survey of programs: Findings from 2014*. San Francisco: Global Health Group, Global Health Sciences, University of California.

Chapter 5
Review of Research Studies

Abstract In this chapter, we discuss peer-reviewed as well as other available research studies on quality of care in family planning in India. We have classified research studies in one or more of the following categories depending upon their major focus: status of quality of care; interventions to improve quality of care; factors influencing quality of care; and impact of improved quality of care. Evidence-based interventions to accelerate improvements in quality of care need to be implemented through an appropriate research agenda to enhance progress towards realizing India's family planning programme goals.

Keywords Evidence based · Informed choice · Reproductive rights Factors influencing quality · Impact of quality of care

5.1 Introduction

In this chapter, we discuss peer-reviewed as well as other available research studies on QoC in FP in India. In 1994, the International Conference on Population and Development was organized in Cairo, and this conference upheld the principle of "reproductive rights". Central to the conference resolutions was the concept of voluntary informed choice and the importance of providing information and services to all individuals and couples (UN 2016).

The ICPD changed the discourse on FP. Therefore, we begin with a review of QoC based on a workshop held in 1995 by Koenig and Khan (1999). We could find only a very few studies in the published literature. Our discussions with key informants did not provide many new leads on researches. The literature that we could access is summarized under the following four categories:

1. Status of QoC provided: what is the QoC that is delivered
2. Interventions to improve QoC: evaluations of interventions and their scale-up
3. Factors influencing QoC: insights providing deeper understanding, which may lead to formulating innovative interventions
4. Impact of improved QoC: consequences of different levels of QoC delivered.

5.2 Review of Quality of Care Around 1994

A workshop held in 1995 on "The Quality of Services in the Indian Family Planning Programme" brought together diverse stakeholders including researchers, policy makers, NGOs, public health physicians, social scientists, and women's health activists (Koenig and Khan 1999). The participants at this meeting reviewed QoC from four perspectives: clients' perspectives, providers' perspectives, QoC in sterilization camps, and programmatic and policy issues associated with improving QoC. Below, we briefly summarize the findings.

5.2.1 Clients' Perspectives

Quality of care concerns among two northern (Bihar and West Bengal) and two southern states (Karnataka and Tamil Nadu) were almost similar although their contraceptive prevalence varied widely—dominant emphasis on sterilization, limited information to clients on method use and side effects (Roy and Verma 1999).

Workers may make selective decisions about providing contraceptive choice and information, with women residing in more remote communities and poorer women substantially less likely to have been informed about spacing methods of contraception and method side effects (Murthy 1999).

In some difficult settings in Uttar Pradesh, north India, programme outreach was found to be limited. Although women had favourable views about services they received, many were reluctant to recommend sterilization or IUD to others, perhaps not surprising in view of the significant rates of method-related complications and low levels of follow-up by programme staff after acceptance (Koenig and Khan 1999).

A series of case studies highlighted the important gaps in such service dimensions as voluntary and informed contraceptive choice, and the technical standards and competence of programme staff in Tamil Nadu (Sundari 1999).

Observation of client–provider interaction in Madhya Pradesh highlighted the systemic problems of access and quality due to infrequent outreach to remote communities, chronic shortages of equipment and supplies, and an overriding programmatic emphasis on sterilization (Barge and Ramachandar 1999).

5.2.2 Provider Perspectives

Despite having the capacity to provide high-quality services in Gujarat, undue emphasis on method-specific targets had detrimental consequences including limited contraceptive choices offered to most long-term method acceptors, the entry of non-health personnel into contraceptive recruitment, and significant over-reporting of acceptance levels for most temporary contraceptive methods (Visaria 1994).

A survey of female paramedical workers in four states (Bihar, West Bengal, Karnataka, and Tamil Nadu) highlight a number of service areas where considerable scope exists for improvement in QoC in contraceptive information and choice, technical competence, and follow-up (Roy and Verma 1999).

Studies in Karnataka and Maharashtra found that providers face considerable barriers in providing reasonable standards of care to clients, including non-residence of providers, inadequate infrastructure, chronic shortages of key medicines and supplies, and difficulties in outreach (Bhatia 1999; Iyer and Jesani 1999).

Sterilization camps were a primary source of clinical contraceptive services in much of rural India. Studies conducted around 1995 in several states highlight QoC concerns, although the capacity of such camps to offer high standards of care appears to vary by location, with the QoC most problematic in outreach settings. Although surgeons are well trained, there were shortcuts in the sterilization of surgical equipment and instruments and in overall infection control measures, major shortcomings in client-centred facilities including unclean toilets, lack of running water, lack of privacy and confidentiality, little pre-operative counselling, and inadequate post-operative recovery facilities (Gupta and Ramanathan 1995; Mavalankar and Sharma 1999; Barge and Ramachandar 1999; Townsend and Khan 1999).

5.2.3 Improving Quality of Care

One intervention at the field level by an NGO, ARCH, in Gujarat showed that educating clients on reproductive anatomy, demonstrating how IUDs work, addressing women's fears and concerns through counselling, and providing information on method complications resulted in significant reductions in IUD dropout rates (Patel and Mehta 2003).

Satia and Sokhi (1999) argue for substituting method-specific targets with other strategic drivers—indicators that provide the driving force for the overall programme. Potential alternative programme drivers include increased access and availability of client services, better performance and coverage, and higher QoC and/ or impact indicators. Requisite changes in supervisory and management information systems would be required to accompany the changes in programme drivers.

5.3 Studies Since 1995 on the Quality of Care Provided

Thus, in 1995, major issues in QoC were: limited information to clients on methods and their use as well as providers making selective choices for clients limiting their informed choice; technical competence; and inadequate follow-up. Some of the deficiencies in QoC were due to inadequate facilities, equipment, and supplies.

After signing the Programme of Action of the ICPD (PoA-ICPD 1994), the Government of India made many changes in the way the FP programme was designed and implemented. It removed all administratively determined targets, and the so called target-free approach was instituted. Method-specific targets were abandoned, and standard operating procedures and QA mechanisms were introduced.

In 1997, the government launched the new reproductive and child health programme, replacing the much narrower programmes on maternal and child health and FP. Koenig et al. (2000) review evidence on QoC within the Indian programme. The review highlights the serious and systemic shortcomings in QoC that characterize the Indian programme in such areas as restricted method choice, limited information provided to the clients, poor technical standards, and low levels of follow-up and continuity of care. Koenig et al. comment:

> These policies aimed at fundamentally reorienting the family planning programme toward a client-centered approach represent positive and long overdue changes, and are likely to have a positive impact in those areas of India where the programme is fully operational. At the same time, it is important to recognize that by themselves, these policy changes fail to redress systemic and complex problems of implementation which continue to plague much of the Indian program. As our review has highlighted, many of these problems defy simple or ready interventions. As such, reorienting Indian family planning services toward a higher quality, more client-centered approach represents a formidable task. Progress toward this end is likely to prove painstakingly slow, and will require an extended timeframe measured more in decades than in years.

The National Population Policy, 2000, utilized the principles of the Cairo conference. Even though the Government of India shifted its programme focus from female sterilization to an approach focusing on birth spacing and temporary methods, sterilization continued to be the mainstay of the programme. India being a large county, the programmes delivered on the ground can be very different from policy intentions.

5.4 Status of Quality of Care

Several measures have been taken by the government and NGOs to improve QoC, as discussed in the previous two chapters. As subsequent studies discussed below show, however, despite several measures and improvements, QoC issues persist. The pace of improvement in QoC has been very gradual. For instance, the percentage of users ever told about the side effects of the current method increased from 34.4% in NFHS-3 (2005–2006) to 46.5% in NFHS-4 (2015) in India, a modest increase of 12 points over a decade.

In a survey in 1998 (NFSH-2), all the interviewed women were asked about the home visits of health workers during the past 12 months, followed by the frequency of visits, and different matters relating to RCH services. The survey showed that only 13% of women age 15–49 in India had received a home visit by a health worker preceding the survey.

Healthwatch, an NGO network, conducted a study on 10 RCH camps in the state of Uttar Pradesh during 2002–2003 (Das et al. 2004). A checklist-cum-questionnaire was prepared based on the MoHFW guidelines. The QoC varied among camps. However, there were no private spaces for counselling and women were not informed about other methods. Several shortfalls in adherence to technical protocols were observed and physical facilities were often inadequate. Infection practices needed to be strengthened. Researchers recommended wider dissemination of standards of care, and that the complications of sterilization should be addressed. They argued that "the poor quality of care that women receive in tubectomy camps in Uttar Pradesh translates into a heavy burden of failure, morbidity and often mortality. There is an urgent need to ensure that standards of care are implemented and some form of redressal mechanism established." The network filed a writ petition in the Supreme Court, and the court passed orders in 2005 for improving the QoC in sterilization operations, including an indemnity scheme, and establishment of QA mechanisms (Chap. 3).

In a subsequent study in 2008 on whether the Supreme Court guidelines had made a difference, researchers reviewed QoC at 17 sterilization camps across the states of Bihar, Uttar Pradesh, Odisha, Jharkhand, and Rajasthan (Chowdhury et al. 2010). The study used a mix of methods including observation of camps and interviews with women as well as providers and district and state officials. The overall message of this study is that there has been a significant improvement in QoC in sterilization services through camps. However, there are still gaps in the implementation of quality standards and monitoring mechanisms. Some of the crucial areas of quality that continued to be ignored are counselling, pre-operative screening procedures as well as post-operative procedures, and discharge-related advice. The clients were neither informed about the insurance scheme nor were they encouraged to file insurance claims in cases of failures or complications.

Pal et al. (2009–10), in their assessment of QoC in female sterilization in one block of Bundi district in Rajasthan, noted that about half the women received "poor" health care services (score 12 or less out of 28), while another 45% received "average" quality of sterilization health care services (score between 13 and 17 out of 28). They found that a clear relationship existed between the quality of health care service and the incidence of adverse health outcomes, with 72% of the women who had received "poor" health care service reporting at least one adverse health outcome subsequently.

Recently, an assessment was conducted of QoC in provision of female sterilization services in 79 public and private facilities in five districts of Bihar—Katihar, Nawada, Purvi Champaran, Samastipur, and Rohtas (Achyut et al. 2016). This study used multiple data collection tools—facility audits, interviews with health care providers and interviews with women who had been sterilized the previous week. It found that, despite a commitment to provide high-quality services, gaps in QoC, although variable, remain. The gaps in the facilities include a lack of qualified staff, few safe spaces for women to discuss questions or concerns about their RH, missing necessary post-operative drugs, as well as infection control. Only a few facilities had the minimum required supply of drugs and equipment to effectively provide sterilization services. A majority of clients were not knowledgeable about contraception beyond sterilization—only 30% had used any method before. Women were motivated and came forth for sterilization, but the level of pre-surgery counselling and care given at the facility was minimal. Very little information was provided about minor problems after surgery and medical conditions which may require a revisit to the facility. Regarding patient satisfaction, the study concluded that a majority of the women reported that providers were friendly; expressed their intent to revisit the facility; and said they would recommend it to others. But they also suggested that cleanliness, waiting time, and care by doctors needed to be improved. The assessment emphasized the need to bridge the gaps in QoC in service delivery, including building the gender perspectives of health providers along with technical competencies. Community mobilization is needed to enable the community to demand for quality of care and make the system more accountable.

The deaths of 13 women operated on at a sterilization camp at Bilaspur, Chhattisgarh, in 2015 was widely reported in media as well as commented upon in research journals (BMJ 2014; Lancet 2014). Das and Contractor (2014) argue that QoC has taken a back seat despite guidelines and QACs and insurance mechanisms. An assessment by the PFI highlights that the Government of India must adhere to its commitment to informed free choice and not impose targets or any form of coercion in the FP programme. More specifically, the report recommends the following:

1. Discontinue incentives for all service providers.
2. Promote spacing methods like oral pills, condoms, IUCDs, and add new methods.
3. Stop sterilization targets as well as sterilization in camps.
4. Carry out FP services on fixed days.
5. Plan and orient all officials at the block, district, and state levels on sterilization procedures and QA.
6. Fill all posts of doctors lying vacant in the state and train more doctors in sterilization procedures in the state.
7. Strengthen the drug procurement policy.

Media reports highlight the need for improving QoC in sterilization procedures. Twenty-six deaths following female sterilization were reported during five years in Mumbai, where over 100,000 successful surgeries were carried out (Debroy 2016). Health officials mentioned that in most cases of deaths, women had underlying health complications that worsened soon after the sterilization procedure.

To assess informed choice and QoC in FP counselling, simulated client interviews were used (León et al. 2007). The simulated client methodology reliably measures QoC in FP. In this technique, trained clients enact a specific client profile, receive services, observe provider behaviour, and report their observations. This study compares results from simulated client visits in three countries—India, Peru, and Rwanda—and discusses the lessons learned from the application of this methodology in diverse settings. Specifically, the thoroughness and neutrality of providers offering DMPA, sterilization, the standard days method, and oral contraceptives were assessed to provide a reliable measurement of informed choice and QoC. Results of simulated client interviews in India (81), Peru (62), and Rwanda (43) revealed that providers scored high on interpersonal relations, but based counselling on medical issues, ignoring reproductive intentions and partner cooperation. Information exchanged on the method chosen, such as side effects, was scarce. Few discussed condom use, despite client need. In Peru, less than 5% of DMPA clients received condom information. Trends were similar across countries, although quality varied significantly. Peruvian providers scored significantly higher than Indian providers, with mean scores of 30 versus 14 for pill clients. Counselling duration was longer in Peru, averaging 17 min versus 10 min in India. Providers obtained higher scores for the predominant programme method, for example, sterilization in India.

5.5 Informed Choice and Discontinuation Rates

While research attention has been directed towards QoC received by women for sterilization, with particular focus on the technical aspects, informed choice and information exchanged between service providers and women have received little attention. Jain (2016) analyses information about methods received by contraceptive users in India based on NFHS-3 (2005–2006 data). He finds that contraceptive users are getting very little information about the method they are using. For example, only 14% of users reported receiving information on all three to four items, such as side effects associated with the method, how to manage them, and about another method. This low level is prevalent across different segments of the society and across all the major states. There are a few exceptions, but the level is still quite low.

The data on women using pills, IUD, injectables, or sterilization captured in NFHS-3 and on those who had started using a method within the previous five years was analysed. These women were asked whether or not at that time (when they started using the method) they were told about the side effects of the method they currently used, how to manage these side effects, or about another method. In addition, women who were sterilized were also asked whether or not they were told that sterilization is permanent.

About 50% of IUD users reported receiving information on each of these three items. Between 25 and 30% of sterilized women reported receiving information about these three items. In addition, about one in three sterilized women reported that they were not told that the method was permanent. A total information index was constructed based upon answers to these questions, which could range from 0 to 100. The value of this method information index for all women and methods combined was very low at only 14.5%, which means that a small number of women (one in six) reported receiving information on all items. Moreover, this level was found to be uniformly low in all strata of the society, including pill, injectables, and sterilization users.

Method information can help improve continuation rates. The one-year discontinuation rate was high—about 42% for modern reversible methods. Discontinuation of injectables was the highest (53%) followed by the pill (49%), condoms (45%), and IUD (20%). Only 1 out of 10 users switched to another method after discontinuation. This survey further documented that about 22% of women in India had an unmet need for contraception in 2005–2006. Past users in India who continue to have an unmet need in the present contributed 27% to this current unmet need. Continuation of the high discontinuation rate of contraception in the future is likely to contribute another 10% of current users to unmet need (Jain 2016).

In order to improve continuity of contraceptive use, clients need to be told about the possibility of switching to another method or service delivery point for obtaining supply of methods. This type of information will help to reassure women that method switching is an acceptable option whenever the original method does not remain suitable for them (e.g., the experience of side effects), or when their reproductive needs and circumstances change. This will inevitably improve the continuity of contraceptive use, irrespective of the method used.

Based upon this analysis, Jain (2016) recommends that MoHFW include this critical component of quality and places greater emphasis on improving quality of services in the country. In the case of sterilization, the doctor, before s/he makes an incision, must ask a few questions, especially regarding whether the woman wants to stop childbearing completely, whether she knows that the operation is permanent, whether she has tried any other method. In addition, s/he must tell the woman about the possible side effects of the operation, and how to manage them if they occur.

Discontinuation rates of contraceptive methods have not received much research attention in India, although one in five contraceptive users use a temporary method. Barden-O'Fallon et al. (2014) analyse panel data on 4000 non-sterilized women at baseline in 2010, and a follow-up survey in 2012 in four cities of Uttar Pradesh. The group of multiple method users was small in comparison to the groups of women using a single method throughout the calendar period. This indicates that there was little method switching between condoms, traditional methods, and other forms of modern methods reported in the calendar. The research findings suggest the need for improving QoC to address unmet need, as method-related reasons accounted for nearly half (47.6%) of the first discontinuation. Improved access to a full array of methods and knowledge of the method's true side effects are needed to ensure that women select the best method suited to their needs. All women should understand the concept of method switching, how to change methods effectively and avoid unwanted pregnancies. Only 2.6% of the women had used more than one temporary method. Thus, there is a need to address women's health concerns and fear of side effects.

5.6 Service Quality for Adolescent and Young People

Shireen et al. (2014) find that despite the government's attempts to provide adolescent-friendly health services through special clinics, they have limited coverage. Through surveys around selected adolescent-friendly clinics, researchers found that young women were more likely to seek help than young men, and married women were more likely to seek help than unmarried women; but that a pervasive lack of trust in the health system stopped many young people from seeking professional help when they had concerns. The quality of services received by clients at these clinics in their experience was mixed. Most clients were able to consult a health care provider, were confident about confidentiality, and were treated fairly. However, clients also reported that there was lack of privacy, and providers, at times, were judgemental. Health services were not the preferred source of information.

Providers (ASHAs, ANMs, counsellors, and medical officers) were also surveyed in these three states—Jharkhand, Maharashtra, and Rajasthan. Generally, providers had received basic training in adolescent RH, mainly covering issues such as nutrition and menstrual hygiene, but lacked training on contraception, sexuality, and pregnancy. They also lacked training in non-judgemental communication methods. Although most providers believed that young people should learn about these aspects, generally only married young people received counselling on these topics, and providers reported that most of the interactions with clients break down along gendered lines. Providers also reported that they could provide quality SRH services if they had better training. Researchers recommended action to increase awareness and availability of services as well as improve the quality of services provided at these clinics.

5.7 Intervention to Improve Quality of Care

We found that the research literature on interventions to improve QoC is particularly sparse, although many interventions have been made, as presented in Chaps. 3 and 4, and, of these, a high proportion have been evaluated. These interventions generally focus on specific components such as counselling or training of providers. We will not repeat their results here. Instead, below we discuss the results of interventions to improve QoC in the published literature.

Programme actions to provide additional inputs in terms of physical facilities, staffing, training, and equipment have some impact on maternal health care, but service delivery still remains far from optimal. Unfortunately, a similar analysis is not available for FP. Similarly, providing counsellors at facilities increased the satisfaction of clients with the information they received, as well as leading to increased use of contraception. However, the health system setting in which these counsellors worked limited their potential impact. There is weak evidence that interventions for engaging men and improving gender equity attitudes improve QoC. It is not clear whether sharing findings from community monitoring in public fora had any impact, but social audit led to legal action and the institution of indemnity schemes for deaths and failures from sterilization as well as the setting up of QA cells and committees for sterilization. Introducing DMPA in the private sector led to expansion of choice and improved QoC, but its use remained limited. Much more research is needed to identify what mix of interventions can remedy gaps in QoC.

5.7.1 *Facility-Level Interventions*

The NRHM accorded due recognition to QoC at the policy and planning levels, and provided additional inputs in terms of physical facilities, staffing, training, and equipment. Examining the available evidence on impact of NRHM on QoC in maternal health care, Nair and Panda (2011) found that quality is a more significant predictor of utilization of maternal health care than access. They found that there has been some improvement in the quality of maternal health services, but it is still a long way off from the standards of care in most emerging economies. There is a need to improve facilities and provide a friendly environment to clients.

The Government of Bihar has placed 105 counsellors in selected high-volume facilities. They have been trained and provided counselling kits and reporting formats. The supervision is provided by the gynaecological and obstetric department of the facility. An evaluation study showed that 79% of the clients had come for counselling services and 21% for a pregnancy test or for antenatal care. Ten per cent of the clients had used a contraceptive earlier. After the appointment of counsellors, coverage by counselling services has increased. Seventy-seven per cent of the clients in facilities with counsellors were counselled on FP methods, whereas only 29% were so counselled in facilities without counsellors. The follow-up with clients showed that a higher proportion of clients who were counselled used contraceptives compared to those who were not. Almost all clients were satisfied with the counselling services, and most of them found the information they received useful. Counsellors' presence had increased the number of FP acceptors—four facilities reported up to a 25% increase, five reported an increase between 40 and 50%, and one above 60%. Thus, FP counsellors had played an important role. However, several challenges need to be addressed for full realization of their potential, including infrastructural inadequacy, indifference towards the importance of counselling by hospital authorities, operational challenges, and counsellors being assigned multifarious responsibilities (Pandey 2016).

5.7.2 Programme-Level Interventions

It is well established that adding new methods to a programme and expanding choice improves QoC and continuation of DMPA, an injectable contraceptive. Although approved for use in private sector, it was not approved for public sector provision until recently. The Dimpa programme has been implemented by Abt Associates over a period of 12 years, and has achieved significant improvement in access, quality, demand for, and use of DMPA.

Can demand generation activities improve QoC? In India, UHI implemented demand creation activities in addition to strengthening service delivery (see Chap. 3; Fotso et al. 2013). Demand creation activities included interpersonal communication, mass media (radio and television), and some mid-media activities. The research based on a two-year mid-line concluded that demand generation activities that were significantly associated with increased use of modern contraception included: (*a*) community outreach activities, such as home visits and group discussions about FP; (*b*) local radio and television programmes; and (*c*) branded slogans and print materials circulated widely across the city. Exposure to more media activities may increase women's likelihood of using contraception. Although dialogues about FP and media activities included knowledge and perceptions of FP methods, it is not clear to what extent choice increased and these activities helped improve method knowledge. In addition, short-term changes in quality and access to FP services may have influenced the results. In India, more than 40% of women recalled exposure to a UHI television programme, whereas 23% reported exposure to a community health worker and only 5% to a UHI radio programme.

5.7.3 Community-Level Interventions

Speizer et al. (2014) evaluated a project which recruited and trained male community health workers to complement the work of ASHAs in a rural district in Odisha. The qualitative research, albeit with very small sample, showed that male engagement can improve delivery, access, and uptake of MNCH services in the context of prevailing gender norms and gender roles in rural India. The study unveiled the complementarity of male and female community health workers in the community-based delivery of, and increased demand for, MNCH services.

Counselling Husbands to Achieve RH and M Equity (CHARM) was a gender equity and FP intervention for men and couples in rural Maharashtra. It sought to increase male engagement through gender equity counselling and greater focus on spacing contraception (Yore et al. 2016). The project involved outreach and intervention by local village health providers. For this study, a multi-session intervention delivered to men but inclusive of their wives was developed and evaluated as a two-armed cluster randomized controlled design study conducted across 50 mapped clusters in rural Maharashtra. Eligible rural young husbands and their wives ($n = 1081$) participated in a three-session FP programme focused on gender equity, delivered to the men (sessions 1 and 2) and their wives (session 3) by village health providers in rural India. Survey assessments were conducted at baseline and at 9- and 18-month follow-ups with eligible men and their wives, and pregnancy tests were obtained from wives at baseline and 18-month follow-up. Additional in-depth understanding of how intervention impact occurred was assessed via in-depth interviews at the 18-month follow-up with village health providers and a sub-sample of couples ($n = 50$, two couples per intervention cluster). Process evaluation was conducted to collect feedback from husbands, wives, and village health providers on programme quality and to ascertain whether programme elements were implemented according to curriculum protocols. Fidelity to intervention protocol was assessed via review of clinical records. The study found that there was positive response in terms of young men recruited for participation. The procedures were implemented with no adverse events and with good participation in the CHARM intervention (91.3% of men received at least one session) and strong evaluation follow-up (>80% retention at each follow-up).

Community-based monitoring of the FP programme in 50 villages of 10 districts in Uttar Pradesh and Bihar highlight concerns related to lack of care and informed choice (Phukan 2015). This experience suggests accountability issues and challenges in terms of gaps in service delivery of FP. The entire process of community-based monitoring was led by women selected and trained from the community in villages. Community meetings and focus group discussions were held in each village. Interviews were conducted with women users of contraception. Data was also collected from service providers under themes like knowledge of FP methods, counselling provided, options available, preparedness of facility, quality of clinical services, follow-up and management, and targets given (if any). The findings from client discussions showed that:

- the focus was on limiting methods with neglect of spacing methods, particularly for method-specific counselling;
- counselling on side effects, method use of OCP, and follow-up were poor; and
- some technical procedures were shortchanged such as pelvic examination before insertion of IUD.

Provider discussions and facility visits to the PHC/CHC showed that:

- There were shortfalls in staff, equipment, and supplies of contraceptives for providing FP services.
- The informal system of targets for sterilization was still in vogue.

Even though findings were shared in public dialogues including providers, it was not clear what actions were taken.

In 2000, a group of activists of the Health Watch Group realized that there was no data on failures and complications after sterilization in the state of Uttar Pradesh. The group mobilized other NGOs who felt that this was a serious case of failure of reproductive rights, and agreed to document cases of complications, failures, and deaths using a case study format. After completion of case studies, a public hearing was held. Despite mobilizing a large number of organizations and media persons, the hearing did not elicit a response from the government. Subsequently, the group evaluated sterilization camps using a checklist derived from government guidelines (see section on status of FP in this chapter). Observations of camps showed that guidelines were not being followed fully. The group, in collaboration with a rights group, filed a public interest litigation in the Supreme Court in 2003. In 2005, the Supreme Court not only passed orders for a stricter compliance mechanism relating to QoC in operations, but also directed the government to institute a national insurance policy to cover all persons undergoing sterilization operations. In November 2005, the Government of India initiated the Family Insurance Scheme and started the QA mechanism in all districts for monitoring FP operations (see Chap. 3). Subsequently, the QA mechanism was extended to all RH services under NRHM across all states.

5.8 Factors Influencing Quality of Care

Several factors affect QoC in FP. However, our understanding of the effect of these factors remains rather limited. On the service delivery side, better access to a health facility within the village has a positive influence, whereas provider biases detract from choice. Ignorance and fear, negative attitudes towards male sterilization, and gender-inequitable roles have an adverse influence on QoC. Higher aspiration for children and media exposure for literate women seem to have a positive influence on QoC.

Thus, provider values and norms as direct proximate variables, and access to facilities as an indirect proximate variable, have been found to have some influence. Distal variables having a direct effect on QoC that have been studied are agency and autonomy of clients as well as community values and norms. We need to have a deeper understanding of the effect of the health system and social environment in which providers function, as well as of the political and legal context of the health system, on QoC in FP.

Reflecting on women's perceptions of their unmet need for FP, Yinger (1998) raises questions regarding the concept and measurement of unmet need, arguing that ignorance and fear cloud major reproductive events for women and men, that ignorance and fear should not be equated with stupidity, and that socio-cultural barriers are formidable but not insurmountable. Nine policy questions evolved from the findings of a three-year ICRW study by Yinger (1998) in Guatemala, India, and Zambia to determine women's perspectives of unmet need for FP in order to improve the standard definition used in demographic and health surveys. The questions were the following: (1) How can FP programmes better help people make informed choices about their reproductive lives? (2) How do people's attitudes towards FP affect unmet need? (3) How can efforts to address unmet need benefit from a better understanding of sex behaviour? (4) How can socio-cultural barriers to

FP be addressed by RH programmes? (5) What is the relationship between QoC and unmet need? (6) Can lowering barriers to effective use of FP be an indicator of progress? (7) Should the definition of unmet need be modified to reflect the risks of unintended pregnancy instead of just the risk from non-use of FP? (8) and (9) Do other policy-relevant ways exist to reflect the heterogeneity of women defined to have unmet need, and how can service delivery be improved by moving from a standardized definition of unmet need to a standardized process that asks the right questions?

Investigating factors affecting the acceptance of vasectomy in the state of Uttar Pradesh, Scott et al. (2011), using qualitative research, found that both men and women reported negative attitudes towards vasectomy, sharing many stories of times when the procedure had not worked or had resulted in physical weakness, thus limiting a man's ability to provide for his family. Female sterilization, on the other hand, was widely accepted and common. The key driver for a man to accept vasectomy was the wife being seen as too weak or sick, and the decision being taken without consulting the wife or the mother. Worry about NSV's impact on men's performance emerged as another barrier. Fear of failure of the procedure itself was found to be a notable barrier to NSV acceptance. A programme to promote NSV will need to address both method-related and socio-cultural barriers including myths and misconceptions about NSV.

A study by Pandey et al. (2013) of the correlation between different factors affecting contraceptive use in Uttarakhand showed that sterilization use was greater among women with good socio-economic conditions as compared to their poorer counterparts. The different factors which are positively associated with sterilization are: membership in a rural women's group, met desire for sons and daughters, educational aspirations for sons and daughters, desire to have a house, and perceived economic constraints in having children.

Using data from NFHS-1 (1992–1993) and NFHS-2 (1998–1999), Dwivedi and Sundaram (2001) conclude that more than half the change in contraceptive behaviour can be explained by increase in propensity to use contraception among illiterate women and women who have a health facility within the village. Media exposure among educated women contributes more towards contraceptive adoption than among illiterate women.

Providers may impose restrictions on clients' access to FP, thus adversely affecting informed choice. In a mixed-method study in Uttar Pradesh, Calhoun et al. (2013) showed that providers restrict clients' access to spacing and long-acting permanent methods of FP based on age, parity, partner consent, and marital status. Qualitative research reinforced the findings that providers, at times, make judgements about their clients' education, FP needs, and ability to understand FP options, thereby imposing unnecessary barriers to access to FP methods. These findings highlight the need for in-service training for staff with a focus on reviewing current guidelines and eligibility criteria for provision of methods. The study found that gender norms and cultural practices affect providers' attitudes and counselling behaviour, so that undereducated, poor, and newlywed women were less likely to receive FP counselling by a provider in the urban Uttar Pradesh sites studied.

In a village in Maharashtra, Wasnik et al. (2013) find that the reasons for the unmet need for contraception were lack of knowledge, health concerns, and religious beliefs. Anand et al. (2010) find that fear of side effects accounted for nearly half of the current need among married women attending immunization clinics in a hospital in Punjab, while the remaining women perceived low risk of pregnancy. However, the women also mentioned opposition from husbands/families, son preference, and lack of inter-spousal communication as reasons for non-use of contraception.

Brault et al. (2016) study multi-level perspectives in low-income communities in Mumbai. They find that FP policies, socio-economic factors, and gender roles constrain women's reproductive choices. They find shortfalls in QoC in provision of sterilization. Procedures for sterilization rarely follow protocol fully, particularly during pre-procedure counselling and consent. Women who chose sterilization often marry early, begin conceiving soon after marriage, and reach or exceed family size early due to problems in accessing reversible contraceptives. Despite these constraints, this study indicates that from the perspective of women, the decision to undergo sterilization is empowering, as they have fulfilled their reproductive duties and can effectively exercise control over their fertility and sexuality. This empowerment results in little post-sterilization regret, improved emotional health, and improved sexual relationships following sterilization.

Mishra et al. (2014), based upon data from selected cities in Uttar Pradesh, find that most men have a high or moderate level of gender-sensitive decision making, have a low to moderate level of restriction on their wife's mobility, and have a moderate to high level of gender-equitable attitudes. As men play a crucial role in contraceptive decision making, this study demonstrates the need to engage men and address gender-equitable attitudes.

Based on a descriptive study of the role of household types and household composition on women's RH outcomes, Speizer and Lance (2015) find that more than 93% of the women in their study were either living in their husband's natal home or with their mother-in-law. Both living arrangements do not seem to constrain modern contraceptive use or delivery at an institution.

5.9 Impact of Improved Quality of Care

Improved QoC reduces unmet need through increased acceptance and improved service utilization for contraception as well as reduced discontinuation of contraceptive use. Poor QoC may be suggestive of higher reproductive morbidity of contraceptive users. The adverse effects of unplanned pregnancy on the mother's and child's health due to unmet need for FP remain under-studied and not well appreciated.

Yadav and Dhillon (2015), based on statistical analysis of DLHS-3 (2007–2008) data, assess the role of maternal health service utilization and the role of FP advice provided during antenatal care and postnatal care on FP use and unmet need in Uttar Pradesh. They find that the average treatment effect of all maternal health service utilization on current use of contraception is 3.7%. The effects of receiving FP advice during antenatal and postnatal care are 7.3 and 6.8%, respectively. However, the effect of utilization of maternal health services on reducing unmet need is only 0.5%. Receiving advice during antenatal and postnatal care has led to reduction in unmet need by 3.1 and 1.4%, respectively. Sometimes, increased contraceptive use may not necessarily reduce unmet need if the total demand for limiting and spacing children also simultaneously increases. These findings suggest the need for "effective FP advice" intervention across socio-economic backgrounds.

Does a perceived differential level of QoC affect RH service utilization? A study (Anand and Sinha 2010) in four states—Tamil Nadu, Maharashtra, Bihar, and Jharkhand—showed that doctor availability, waiting time, cleanliness, privacy, and affordability in private health facilities enhance the probability that a health facility will be used for any RH purpose. Medicine availability and treatment effectiveness at the public health facility enhance its service use. The study was mainly secondary and quantitative in nature, and included analysing data collected by the International Institute for Population Sciences and the Johns Hopkins University as a follow-up study to the 1998–1999 NFHS-2. The follow-up survey was carried out in Tamil Nadu, Maharashtra, Bihar, and Jharkhand. In 2002–2003, these four states were selected to capture socio-economic and demographic variations. A scale was constructed to measure utilization levels. Dimensions included service proximity, doctor availability, waiting time, medicines, facility cleanliness, dignified treatment, privacy, service affordability, and treatment effectiveness.

In a study of self-reported morbidity in the context of contraceptive use in a district in Kerala, Sowmini (1999) finds that symptoms suggestive of total reproductive morbidity, reproductive tract infections, and menstrual problems were higher among contraceptive users compared to non-users, which is an argument for improving QoC in contraceptive services.

There is evidence that improved service quality reduces discontinuation of contraceptive use. Two retrospective studies from India suggest a positive link between provision of more intensive counselling and information about method side effects and lower rates of contraceptive discontinuation (Angeles et al. 2001; Bertrand et al. 1996). Poor QoC influences unmet need, which creates a higher probability of resulting in unplanned pregnancy. In a study in India, Singh et al. (2012) found that mistimed pregnancies were positively associated with elevated odds of unsupervised deliveries, incomplete immunization, and post-neonatal mortality. The unwanted pregnancy was associated with neonatal, post-neonatal, and early childhood mortality as well as with stunting and incomplete immunization of the child.

5.10 Research Methodologies Used

Table 5.1 shows the methodologies used by researchers. The status studies have largely relied on mixed methods, and interventions studies have used non-experimental evaluations. We did not find any RCTs (randomized controlled

5.10 Research Methodologies Used

Table 5.1 Research methods used *Source* Authors

Research methodology used	Status	Interventions to improve QoC	Factors affecting QoC	Impact of QoC
Qualitative studies		+	++	
Mixed methods	++++	+	+	+
Data analysis from surveys		+	++++++	+++
Non-experimental evaluations	+	++++++	+	
Case-controlled studies				
Cohort studies				
RCTs				
Systematic reviews/ reviews		+		

trials). Research on both factors affecting QoC and impact of QoC has relied on analysis of data either specially collected or other surveys including the NFHS.

5.11 Global Reviews on Quality of Care in Family Planning

Our review of research studies on QoC in FP are broadly in line with the findings of a recent global review as presented in Table 5.2 (Askew and Brady 2013), as well as discussed below.

Service provision: Clinic-based delivery of FP services is still the main delivery channel for married women. Increasingly, this may be through non-public sector facilities as the private sector grows in many countries. How to provide clinic-based FP services is broadly understood. The evidence shows that primarily the concern is with improving quality and choice.

Status of QoC: Existing evidence indicates that poor-quality counselling and delivery are universal barriers to initiation and sustained use of FP. Limited information to clients on methods constraining their informed choice, lack of technical competence, and inadequate follow-up in India also are QoC issues that persist despite improvements over time.

Interventions to improve QoC: Numerous QI interventions have been developed, but relatively few have been rigorously evaluated (Mwaikambo et al. 2011; RamaRao and Mohanam 2003). The evidence base for which interventions can most efficiently increase the number of methods offered, and which can most effectively improve providers' skills, particularly in counselling new clients to determine and meet their individual needs including continued use of hormonal methods, remains limited, however (Cleland et al. 2006; Halpern et al. 2011; RamaRao and Mohanam 2003). We also found that peer-reviewed published

Table 5.2 A comparison of findings from our review of research studies in india and the global review *Source* Authors

Category	Our review	Global review
Studies on QoC provided	Limited information to clients on methods constraining informed choice, lack of technical competence, and inadequate follow-up in India are QoC issues that persist despite improvements over time	Existing evidence indicates that poor-quality counselling and delivery are universal barriers to initiation and sustained use of FP
Interventions to improve QoC	Peer-reviewed published studies on interventions to improve QoC in India are rather sparse. Much more research is needed to identify what mix of interventions can remedy poor QoC	The evidence base for which interventions can most efficiently increase the number of methods offered, and which can most effectively improve providers' skills, particularly in counselling new clients to determine and meet their individual needs including continued use of hormonal methods, remains limited
Monitoring QoC	Studies on how well QA structures established by government function or rigorous evaluation of their effect on improving QoC are not available	Evidence is also limited regarding the feasibility and effectiveness of QA and monitoring mechanisms
Impact of Improved QoC	Evidence, although limited, indicates that improved QoC reduces unmet need through increased acceptance and improved service utilization for contraception as well as reduced discontinuation of contraceptive use	Substantial evidence exists that strengthening the QoC components in the Bruce-Jain framework does impact client–provider interactions, client satisfaction, and effective and sustained method use

studies on interventions to improve QoC in India are rather sparse. Much more research is needed to identify what mix of interventions can remedy poor QoC.

Monitoring QoC: Evidence is also limited regarding the feasibility and effectiveness of QA and monitoring mechanisms. Several such mechanisms have been piloted over the past two decades, but with little systematic documentation or evaluation. Key issues concerning standardized indicators, data collection systems, and feedback and data utilization mechanisms remain under-researched. In India, investment is needed in generating evidence regarding how such mechanisms can be standardized and function effectively and efficiently. The Indian government has instituted QA mechanisms comprising QACs and QA cells at state and district levels. Limited evidence from one state indicates that they have the potential to improve QoC, but we do not have studies on how well these function, or rigorous evaluation of their effect on improving QoC.

Impact: The key components of high-quality services are well established, as described in the Bruce-Jain framework (Bruce 1990; Jain 2001), and substantial evidence exists that strengthening these components does impact client–provider interactions, client satisfaction, and effective and sustained method use (RamaRao and Mohanam 2003). A recent synthesis of the evidence (Jain and Ross 2012) yielded two broad conclusions: (*a*) increasing the number of methods made available to clients increases choice, which leads to more new users, reduced discontinuation through switching, and increased prevalence overall; and (*b*) improving providers' skills and attitudes enhances their technical competence and ability to identify and meet clients' individual needs.

Research is needed on interventions to improve and sustain the quality of FP services. More evidence is needed to identify feasible and acceptable interventions that enable and require providers to respond to their clients' individual needs. Evidence is also needed regarding their effectiveness and sustainability in both attracting new FP users and in reducing discontinuation, as well as their ability to ensure that the distinct needs of vulnerable and underserved populations are appropriately met. Investment in context-specific operations and implementation research around QI interventions would enable health systems to address the many method- and programme-related factors that are the most commonly cited reasons for non-use of contraception among women with an unmet need.

A key research investment would be the strengthening of QA and monitoring mechanisms to ensure that such improvements are standardized, routinized, and sustained.

Increasing engagement of the commercial sector in providing FP through private clinics is particularly noticeable through the burgeoning of social franchising. Recent reviews (Madhavan and Bishai 2010; Mwaikambo et al. 2011; Stephenson et al. 2012) find strong evidence that franchising does increase access to and use of FP services, moderate evidence of improved quality, and moderate evidence of increased use by the poor. The extent to which franchising addresses equity is, however, uncertain. Only one study has addressed cost-effectiveness, but it was inconclusive. Given the potential of this approach, further research is justified regarding its effect on QoC and equity as well as its relative cost-effectiveness.

5.12 Recent Relevant International Research on Quality of Care

Although our focus in this chapter is on published research results on QoC in FP in India, we discuss below a few relevant recent studies which may have implications for improving QoC in FP in India.

Sustainable development goals offer an opportunity to focus on QoC and re-examine user experiences and their impact on health care utilization. The new framework provides an opening to redress the insidious problem of negative interactions with care across the RMNCH+A services continuum, and to redraft the blueprint for service delivery and performance measurement, placing individuals and their needs at the centre. Both the maternal health and FP fields are at a turning point in their histories of defining and addressing individuals' experiences of care, which includes person-centred care principles, individuals' preferences, needs, and values, and the importance of informed decision making, respect, privacy and confidentiality, and non-discrimination. Promoting respectful, person-centred care also requires recognizing the factors that lead to poor treatment of clients, including gender norms and unsupportive working conditions for providers (Holt et al. 2017). The latest global literature on QoC in FP emphasizes addressing determinants of QoC, such as social norms, provider bias and motivation to provide QoC, counselling to young people, and expanding method choice.

A recent study from Senegal (Assaf et al. 2017) focuses on examining client-centred counselling and provider training as key components of QoC. The study's findings indicate an insufficient level of counselling provided by a low proportion of service providers. Counselling was more likely to be provided to new rather than to returning clients. Clients were significantly less likely to be very satisfied when their providers counselled on side effects and when to return. Clients seen by a provider with FP training had almost twice the odds of having correct knowledge about their method's protection from sexually transmitted infections, compared with clients seen by a provider with no recent training. Another study from Ethiopia (Teshome et al. 2017) concluded that during counselling for FP, women were more likely to report high satisfaction when their provider asked about their partner's attitude towards contraceptive methods and when asked about their concerns and worries regarding FP methods.

Health worker motivation to monitor and optimize contraceptive supply management is a key factor to ensure adequate supply and avoid stock-outs. An intervention (Vermandere et al. 2017) delivered in 15 health facilities in Maputo province, Mozambique, conducted 10 monthly audits to collect data through examination of stock cards and stock counts of six contraceptives. Based on these audits, the two intervention groups received a monthly evaluation report reflecting the quality of their supply management. One of these groups was also awarded material incentives conditional on their performance, and staff motivation was measured through interviewing health care providers. This resulted in enhanced stock management, indicating the importance of feedback for health workers' accomplishment; however, a rise in motivation was not measurable.

Provider bias regarding method appropriateness can restrict people's access to contraceptives. In a study conducted by Schwandt et al. (2017) in urban Nigeria, self-reported biases in service provision (based on age, parity, and marital status) was assessed among providers in health facilities as well as among pharmacists and patent medical vendors in five cities. Minimum age bias was found to be the most common bias, while minimum parity was the least common bias reported by providers. Experience of in-service training for health facility providers was associated with decreased prevalence of marital status bias for the pill, injectable, and IUD; however, training experience did not have any effect, or had the opposite effect on, pharmacists' and patent medical vendor operators' reports of service provision bias. Study results suggest developing interventions for youth which aim at increasing supportive provision of contraceptives and addressing provider biases in service provision. In addition, it is also important to understand users' attitudes towards or experiences with provider influence and bias regarding contraception.

Higgins et al. (2016) conducted a study among young adult women with any history of contraceptive use to address the gap in provider bias in promoting reversible contraception. Women often described providers as a trusted source of contraceptive information; however, several women reported that their preferences regarding contraceptive selection or removal were not considered. Many participants believed that providers recommend long-acting reversible contraception (LARC) disproportionately to socially marginalized women. The study encourages following contraceptive counselling and removal protocols that directly address reproductive injustices and that respect patients' wishes.

Another study from Mozambique (Chavane et al. 2017) conducted exit interviews to assess women's satisfaction with FP services. The survey, conducted in 174 health facilities, was representative at the national level, covered all provinces, and both urban and rural areas. Overall, 86% of respondents were satisfied with FP services, but issues such as insufficient supplies of oral contraceptives and the low quality of health care and provider–client interactions were given as reasons for women's dissatisfaction. Thus, the study suggests that defined actions at the level of health service provision are needed to tackle the identified issues and ensure improved satisfaction with, and better utilization of, FP services.

Communication and interpersonal skills are increasingly emphasized in the measurement of health care quality, yet there is limited research on the association of interpersonal care with health outcomes. Dehlendorf et al. (2016) conducted a study on patient–provider communication to determine whether the quality of interpersonal care during contraceptive counselling is associated with contraceptive use over time, using a prospective cohort study of 348 women. The study provides evidence that the quality of interpersonal care, measured using both patient reports and observation of provider behaviours, influences contraceptive use, thus supporting attention to interpersonal communication as an important aspect of health care quality. The associations of establishing rapport and eliciting the patient perspective with contraceptive continuation are suggestive of the areas of focus for provider communication skills training for contraceptive care.

Demand generation for FP is one of the strategies to improve uptake and use of contraception, as an essential complement to policies and supply-side interventions. However, there is a need to synthesize evidence on the impacts and costs of FP demand generation interventions and on their effectiveness in improving modern contraceptive use, and to identify the indicators used to assess effectiveness, cost-effectiveness, and impacts of demand generation interventions (Belaid et al. 2015).

Socio-cultural norms and male participation play a major role in FP decision making. There is a need to examine the role of socio-cultural inhibitions in the use of modern contraceptives. Socio-cultural expectations and values attached to marriage, women, and childbearing remain an impediment to using FP methods. For example, men have an important role to play towards acceptance of FP methods; thus, programme efforts often identify strategies to engage men in FP services. However, it is important to determine the extent to which men accept these interventions.

A cross-sectional study by Msovela and Tengia-Kessy (2016) was conducted in Kenya among 365 currently married or cohabiting couples who had at least one child under the age of 5 years. The study found that men were engaged in FP services through their spouses, either verbally or by using partner notification cards, incorporating FP messages during monthly meetings and community outreach programmes. Although these strategies have been shown to encourage men to engage in FP services, these interventions reach few men, and hence there is a need to scale up programme strategies to improve uptake of FP services. In Burkina Faso, the combination of local culture and community participation is seen as an effective approach to reducing cultural barriers of access to health services, including FP. These events helped reduce the negative impact of perceptions, inaccurate beliefs, and misinformation about modern contraceptive methods commonly observed in target populations (Kaboré S et al 2016).

Health system strengthening, especially at the facility level, is a policy and programming priority that will contribute to RH and FP for clients, including adolescents. Jayachandran et al. (2016) conducted a study in Malawi to describe the quality, in terms of provision and experience of care, of facility-based FP services for adolescents compared to older clients. Quality of care for adolescents attending facility-based FP services was slightly better than for older clients, but this was overshadowed by the finding of a low standard of care overall.

Sangraula et al. (2017) undertook a QI project to assess QoC before, during, and after LARC services at three school-based health centres in New York City. Although participants were highly satisfied with the LARC services at these school-based health centres, key themes emerged within the domain of communication, such as: balancing the need for information with concerns about being overwhelmed by information; and interest in information that directly addresses misconceptions about LARCs. The study suggested strategies to improve LARC service by providing post-procedure "care packages" with information and supplies, and supporting a peer-based network of adolescent LARC users and previous patients to serve as a resource for new patients. However, the effect of implementing these suggested strategies on reproductive health care use and outcomes is yet to be ascertained.

Masho et al. (2016) conducted a study that highlights the importance of the postpartum care visit in improving modern contraceptive use and guiding health care policy in the effort of reducing unintended pregnancy rates. The study examined the association between postpartum care visit attendance and modern contraceptives by reviewing claims and demographic and administrative data from a managed care organization. Women who attended the postpartum care visit were 50% more likely to use modern contraceptive methods than women who did not.

IntraHealth International applied the "optimizing performance and quality" approach at five health care facilities in Togo, which resulted in significant increases in contraceptive counselling and uptake among post-abortion care clients (Mugore et al. 2016). A baseline assessment identified the following needs: reorganizing services to ensure that contraceptives are provided at point of treatment for abortion complications, before post-abortion care clients are discharged; improving provider competencies in FP services, including in providing LARC implants and IUDs; ensuring that contraceptive methods are available to all post-abortion care clients free of charge; standardizing post-abortion care registers and enhancing data collection and reporting systems; enhancing internal supervision systems at facilities and teamwork among post-abortion care providers; and engaging post-abortion care providers in community talks. This result demonstrates that the solutions applied and devised maintained method choice while expanding access to underused LARCs.

CARE's Supporting Access to Family Planning and Post-abortion Care initiative aims to increase the availability, quality, and use of contraception, with a particular focus on highly effective and full form methods—IUDs and implants—in crisis-affected settings in Chad and the Democratic Republic of the Congo (Rattan et al. 2016). Before the initiative, LARC methods were either unknown or unavailable in the intervention areas. However, as soon as trained providers were in place, they noted a dramatic and sustained increase in new users of all contraceptive methods, especially implants. Key programme modifications included more focused communication through mass media, community, and interpersonal channels about the benefits of IUDs while reinforcing the wide range of methods available, and refresher training for providers on how to insert IUDs to strengthen their competence and confidence. Over time, a gradual redistribution of the method mix was noted in parallel with vigorous continued FP uptake. This experience suggests that analysing the method mix can be helpful for designing programme strategies, and that expanding method choice can accelerate the process of satisfying demand, especially in environments with high unmet need for contraception.

Another study by Darney et al. (2016) examined the associations between age and patient-reported quality of FP services among young women aged 15–29 years in Mexico. The primary outcome was high-quality care, defined as positive responses to all five quality items regarding contraceptive services included in the survey. Adolescents reported a lower quality of FP services compared with young adult women aged 20–24 years and 25–29 years. Self-reported care quality increased for all three age groups between 2006 and 2014. Additionally, the study demonstrated that adolescents who were using hormonal contraception were significantly less likely to respond positively to all five quality items compared with women aged 25–29 years who were using hormonal contraception. Specifically, more adolescents reported not having their concerns about side effects addressed compared with women aged 25–29 years. These findings suggest that gaps exist in the QoC received by adolescents and older women, and there is additional work to be done to meet the needs of adolescents, both to ensure human rights and to prevent unintended pregnancies.

Task shifting from higher-cadre providers to community health workers has been widely adopted to address health care provider shortages, but the addition of any service can potentially add to an already considerable workload for community health workers. Objective measures of workload alone, such as work-related time and travel, may not reflect how community health workers actually perceive and react to their circumstances. Chin-Quee et al. (2016) examine the effect of health workers' perceptions and objective measures of workload on quality of services, performance, and job and client satisfaction in Rwanda. Over 90% of community health workers reported workload manageability, job satisfaction, and motivation to perform their jobs. Clients were highly satisfied with community health worker services, and most stated a preference for future services from community health workers. The study, based on the documented volume of work by community health workers and client perceptions, demonstrated that adding the resupply of hormonal contraceptives to community health workers' tasks would not place an undue burden on them, and would not adversely affect service quality or the relationships between community health workers and clients. Accordingly, the initiative was scaled up in all 30 districts in the country.

In Ethiopia, a community-based cross-sectional study was conducted to understand the determinants of long-acting and permanent contraceptive method use among married women. Survey results showed a significant positive association between utilization of long-acting and permanent contraceptive methods and women's education, women's occupation, number of live children, joint fertility-related decision, having a radio/TV, and discussion with a health care provider about long-acting and permanent contraceptive methods. This highlights the need to aim efforts at women's empowerment, health education, and encouraging open discussion of FP by couples (Melka et al. 2015).

Health behaviours are shaped by *multiple social and environmental factors*. Research on contraceptive uptake has often focused on individual determinants with little attention to community characteristics that may affect access to services and reproductive behaviour. Tappis et al. (2015) studied individual and community determinants of contraceptive use from a cross-sectional survey of 6200 mothers in 503 communities in Sindh, Pakistan. Living in a community where a higher proportion of women received quality antenatal care and where discussion of birth spacing was more common was significantly associated with contraceptive use. Community-wide poverty lowered contraceptive use. Quality of care at the community level has strong effects on contraceptive use, independent of the characteristics of individual households or women. These findings suggest that powerful gains in contraceptive use may be realized by improving the quality of antenatal care, and community health workers should focus on generating discussion of birth spacing in the community.

A study by Campbell et al. (2015) on private sector provision of FP services used 57 nationally representative demographic and health surveys in low- and middle-income countries (2000–2013) in four geographical regions to estimate the need for contraceptive services, and examined the sector of provision, by women's socio-economic position. Modern contraceptive use among women in need was lowest in Sub-Saharan Africa (39%), with the prevalence in other regions ranging from 64 to 72%. The private sector share of the FP market was 37–39% of users across the regions and 37% overall (median across countries: 41%). Private sector users accessed medical providers, specialized drug sellers, and retailers. Private retailers played a more important role in Sub-Saharan Africa (14%) than in other regions (3–5%). Non-governmental organizations and FBOs (Faith Based Organisations) served a small percentage. Privileged women (richest wealth quintile, urban residents, or secondary-/tertiary-level education) used private sector services more than the less privileged. Contraceptive method types with higher requirements (medical skills) for provision were less likely to be acquired from the private sector, while short-acting methods/injectables were more likely. The percentages of women informed of side effects varied by method and provider subtype, but within subtypes they were higher among public than private medical providers for four of five methods assessed. The study concludes that given the importance of private sector providers, there is a need to understand why women choose their services, what quality services the private sector provides, and how it can be improved. However, when prioritizing one of the two sectors (public versus private), it is critical to consider the potential impact on contraceptive prevalence and equity of met need.

It is hypothesized that the *poor quality of FP service provision in many low-income settings is a barrier to contraceptive use.* Tumlinson et al. (2015) used survey data from 3990 women to investigate whether FP service quality was associated with current modern contraceptive use in five cities in Kenya. Audits of selected facilities and service provider interviews were conducted in 260 facilities, and exit interviews were conducted with FP clients at 126 high-volume clinics. Providers' solicitation of clients' method preferences, assistance with method selection, and provision of information on side effects and good treatment of clients were positively associated with current modern contraceptive use (prevalence ratios 1.1 each); associations were often stronger among younger and less educated women. The findings suggest that efforts to assist with method selection and to improve the content of contraceptive counselling and treatment of clients by providers have the potential to increase contraceptive use in urban Kenya.

The above studies reinforce the earlier findings that poor QoC is a barrier to contraceptive use, and person-centred care is an integral part of QoC. Provider biases about method appropriateness among different age groups are a barrier to women receiving QoC. Therefore, client-centred counselling, including for postpartum and post-abortion care; provider training both on technical skills as well as on communication and interpersonal skills; and improving service provision through ensuring adequate supplies and strengthening the health system are required to improve QoC.

Socio-cultural norms and male participation can influence QoC as it is delivered. Ultimately, it should be kept in mind that health behaviours are shaped by multiple social and environmental factors.

References

Achyut, P., Mishra, A., Montana, L., Sengupta, R., Calhoun, L. M., & Nanda, P. (2016). Integration of family planning with maternal health services: An opportunity to increase postpartum modern contraceptive use in urban Uttar Pradesh, India. *Journal of Family Planning and Reproductive Health Care, 42*(2), 107–115. https://doi.org/10.1136/jfprhc-2015-101271.

Anand, B., Singh, J., & Mohi, M. (2010). Study of unmet need for family planning in immunisation clinic of a teaching hospital at Patiala, India. *Internet Journal of Health, 11*(1), 23–24.

Anand, S., & Sinha, R. K. (2010). Quality differentials and reproductive health service utilisation determinants in India. *International Journal of Health Care Quality Assurance, 23*(8), 718–729.

Angeles, G., Dietrich, J., Guilkey, D., Mancini, D., Mroz, T., Tsui, A., et al. (2001). *A meta-analysis of the impact of family planning programs on fertility preferences, contraceptive method choice and fertility*. Washington, D.C.: MEASURE Evaluation, USAID.

Angeles, G., Guilkey, D. K., & Mroz, T. A. (1998). Purposive program placement and the estimation of family planning program effects in Tanzania. *Journal of the American Statistical Association, 93*, 884–899.

Askew, I., & Brady, M. (2013). *Reviewing the evidence and identifying gaps in family planning research: The unfinished agenda to meet FP2020 goals*. Background document for the Family Planning Research Donor Meeting, Washington, D.C., December 3–4, 2012.

Assaf, S., Wang, W., & Mallick, L. (2017). Quality of care in family planning services in Senegal and their outcomes. *BMC Health Services Research, 17*(1), 346. https://doi.org/10.1186/s12913-017-2287-z.

Barden-O'Fallon, J., Speizer, I. S., Calhoun, L. M., Montana, L., & Nanda, P. (2014). Understanding patterns of temporary method use among urban women from Uttar Pradesh, India. *BMC Public Health, 14*, 1018.

Barge, S., & Ramachandar, L. (1999). Provider-client interaction in primary health care: A case study from Madhya Pradesh. In M. A. Koenig & M. E. Khan (Eds.), *Improving quality of care in India's family welfare programme*. New York: Population Council.

Belaid, L., Dumont, A., Chaillet, N., De Brouwere, V., Zertal, A., Hounton, S., et al. (2015). Protocol for a systematic review on the effect of demand generation interventions on uptake and use of modern contraceptives in LMIC. *Systematic Reviews, 4*, 124. https://doi.org/10.1186/s13643-015-0102-7.

Bertrand, J. T., Magnani, R. J., & Rutenberg, N. (1996). *Evaluating family planning programs with adaptations for reproductive health*. Washington, D.C.: The Evaluation Project, USAID.

Bhatia, J.C., & John C. (1999). Health-seeking behaviour of married women and costs incurred: An analysis of prospective data. In S. Pachauri and S. Subramanian (eds), Implementing a reproductive health agenda in India: The beginning. New Delhi: Population Council.

Brault, M. A., Schensul, S. L., Singh, R., Verma, R. K., & Jadhav, K. (2016). Multilevel perspectives on female sterilization in low-income communities in Mumbai, India. *Qualitative Health Research, 26*(11), 1550–1560. https://doi.org/10.1177/1049732315589744.

Bruce, J. (1990). Fundamental elements of the quality of care: A simple framework. *Studies in Family Planning, 21*(2), 61–91.

Calhoun, L. M., Speizer, I. S., Rimal, R., Sripad, P., Chatterjee, N., Achyut, P., et al. (2013). Provider imposed restrictions to clients' access to family planning in urban Uttar Pradesh, India: A mixed methods study. *BMC Health Services Research, 13*, 532. https://doi.org/10.1186/1472-6963-13-532.

Campbell, O. M., Benova, L., Macleod, D., Goodman, C., Footman, K., Pereira, A. L., et al. (2015). Who, what, where: An analysis of private sector family planning provision in 57 low- and middle-income countries. *Tropical Medicine & International Health, 20*(12), 1639–1656. https://doi.org/10.1111/tmi.12597.

Chavane, L., Dgedge, M., Bailey, P., Loquiha, O., Aerts, M., & Temmerman, M. (2017). Assessing women's satisfaction with family planning services in Mozambique. *Journal of Family Planning and Reproductive Health Care, 43*(3), 222–228. https://doi.org/10.1136/jfprhc-2015-101190.

Chin-Quee, D., Mugeni, C., Nkunda, D., Uwizeye, M. R., Stockton, L. L., & Wesson, J. (2016). Balancing workload, motivation and job satisfaction in Rwanda: Assessing the effect of adding family planning service provision to community health worker duties. *Reproductive Health, 13*, 2. https://doi.org/10.1186/s12978-015-0110-z.

References

Chowdhury, J., Lairenlakpam, M., & Das, A. (2010). *Have the Supreme Court guidelines made a difference? A study of quality of care of women's sterilization in five states.* New Delhi: Centre for Health and Social Justice.

Cleland, J., Bernstein, S., Ezeh, A., Faundes, A., Glasier, A., & Innis, J. (2006). Family planning: The unfinished agenda. *Lancet, 368*(9549), 1810–1827.

Darney, B. G., Saavedra-Avendano, B., Sosa-Rubi, S. G., Lozano, R., & Rodriguez, M. I. (2016). Comparison of family-planning service quality reported by adolescents and young adult women in Mexico. *International Journal of Gynecology & Obstetrics, 134*(1), 22–28. https://doi.org/10.1016/j.ijgo.2015.12.003.

Das, A., & Contractor, S. (2014). India's latest sterilisation camp massacre. *BMJ, 349,* g7282. https://doi.org/10.1136/bmj.g7282.

Debroy, S. (2016). 10 dead after female sterilization in 1 year. *Times of India.* http://timesofindia.indiatimes.com/life-style/health-fitness/health-news/10-dead-after-female-sterilization-in-1-year/articleshow/53074269.cms. Accessed January 28, 2018.

Dehlendorf, C., Henderson, J. T., Vittinghoff, E., Grumbach, K., Levy, K., Schmittdiel, J., et al. (2016). Association of the quality of interpersonal care during family planning counseling with contraceptive use. *American Journal of Obstetrics and Gynecology, 215*(1), 78.e1–9. https://doi.org/10.1016/j.ajog.2016.01.173.

Dwivedi, S. N., & Sundaram, K. R. (2001). National family health survey and children. *Indian Journal of Pediatrics, 68*(11), 1047.

Fotso, J. C., Speizer, I. S., Mukiira, C., Kizito, P., & Lumumba, V. (2013). Closing the poor-rich gap in contraceptive use in urban Kenya: Are family planning programs increasingly reaching the urban poor? *International Journal for Equity in Health, 12*(71). https://doi.org/10.1186/1475-9276-12-71.

Halpern, V., Lopez, L. M., Grimes, D. A., & Gallo, M. F. (2011). Strategies to improve adherence and acceptability of hormonal methods of contraception. *Cochrane Database of Systematic Reviews, 4,* CD004317. https://doi.org/10.1002/14651858.cd004317.pub3.

Higgins, J. A., Kramer, R. D., & Ryder, K. M. (2016). Provider bias in long-acting reversible contraception (LARC) promotion and removal: Perceptions of young adult women. *American Journal of Public Health, 106*(11), 1932–1937.

Holt, K., Caglia, J. M., Peca, E., Sherry, J. M., & Langer, A. A. (2017). Call for collaboration on respectful, person-centered health care in family planning and maternal health. *Reproductive Health, 14*(1), 20. https://doi.org/10.1186/s12978-017-0280-y.

Jain, A. (2001). Implications for evaluating the impact of family planning programs with a reproductive health orientation. *Studies in Family Planning, 32*(3), 220–229.

Jain, A. K. (2016). Examining progress and equity in information received by women using a modern method in 25 developing countries. *International Perspectives on Sexual and Reproductive Health, 42*(3), 131–140.

Jain, A. K., Obare, F., RamaRao, S., & Askew, I. (2013). Reducing unmet need by supporting women with met need. *International Perspectives on Sexual and Reproductive Health*, 133–141.

Jain, A. K., RamaRao, S., Kim, J., & Costello, M. (2012). Evaluation of an intervention to improve quality of care in family planning programme in the Philippines. *Journal of Biosocial Science, 44*(1), 27–41. https://doi.org/10.1017/S0021932011000460.

Jain, A. K., & Ross, J. A. (2012). Fertility differences among developing countries: Are they still related to family planning program efforts and social settings? *International Perspectives on Sexual and Reproductive Health, 38*(1), 15–22. https://doi.org/10.1363/3801512.

Jayachandran, V., Chapotera, G., & Stones, W. (2016). Quality of facility-based family planning services for adolescents in Malawi: Findings from a national census of health facilities. *Malawi Medical Journal, 28*(2), 48–52.

Jejeebhoy, S. J., Santhya, K. G., Singh, S. K., et al. (2014). *Provision of reproductive and sexual health services to adolescents and youth in India: The perspectives of health care providers.* New Delhi: Population Council.

Kaboré, S., Savadogo, L. B., Méda, Z. C., Bakouan, K., Lankoandé, E., Zongo, B., et al. (2016). Local culture and community participation: Djandioba family planning day in Burkina Faso. *Sante Publique, 28*(6), 817–826.

Koenig, M. A., & Khan, M. E. (Eds.). (1999). *Improving quality of care in India's family welfare programme*. New York: Population Council.

León, F. R., Lundgren, R., Huapaya, A., Sinai, I., & Jennings, V. (2007). Challenging the courtesy bias interpretation of favorable clients' perceptions of family planning delivery. *Evaluation Review, 31*(1), 24–42.

Madhavan, S., & Bishai, D. (2010). *Private sector engagement in sexual and reproductive health and maternal and neonatal health: A review of the evidence*. London: Department for International Development.

Masho, S. W., Cha, S., Charles, R., McGee, E., Karjane, N., Hines, L., et al. (2016). Postpartum visit attendance increases the use of modern contraceptives. *Journal of Pregnancy*. https://doi.org/10.1155/2016/2058127.

Melka, A. S., Tekelab, T., & Wirtu, D. (2015). Determinants of long acting and permanent contraceptive methods utilization among married women of reproductive age groups in western Ethiopia: A cross-sectional study. *Pan African Medical Journal, 21*, 246. https://doi.org/10.11604/pamj.2015.21.246.5835.

Mishra, S. R., Joshi, M. P., & Khanal, V. (2014). Family planning knowledge and practice among people living with HIV in Nepal. *PLoS ONE, 9*(2), e88663. https://doi.org/10.1371/journal.pone.0088663.

Msovela, J., & Tengia-Kessy, A. (2016). Implementation and acceptability of strategies instituted for engaging men in family planning services in Kibaha district, Tanzania. *Reproductive Health, 13*(1), 138.

Mugore, S., Kassouta, N. T., Sebikali, B., Lundstrom, L., & Saad, A. (2016). Improving the quality of postabortion care services in Togo: Increased uptake of contraception. *Global Health: Science and Practice, 4*(3), 495–505. https://doi.org/10.9745/ghsp-d-16-00212.

Murthy, N. (1999) "The quality of family welfare services in rural Maharashtra: Insights from a client survey," in Improving Quality of Care in India's Family Welfare Programme: The Challenge Ahead,eds.M.A. Koenig and M.E. Khan. New York: Population Council, pp. 33–48.

Mwaikambo, L., Speizer, I. S., Schurmann, A., Morgan, G., & Fikree, F. (2011). What works in family planning interventions: A systematic review. *Studies in Family Planning, 42*, 67–82. https://doi.org/10.1111/j.1728-4465.2011.00267.x.

Nair, H., & Panda, R. (2011). Quality of maternal healthcare in India: Has the National Rural Health Mission made a difference? *Journal of Global Health, 1*, 79–86.

Pandey, S. (2016). *Assessment of efficacy of FP counselors program in Bihar*. Paper presented at the International Conference on Family Planning, Nusa Dua, Indonesia, January 25–28.

Pandey, S., Kannubhai, T. H., Rawat, C. M., Jha, S. K., & Awasthi, S. (2013). Socio-demographic factors influencing family size among rural population of district Nainital, Uttarakhand. *Indian Journal of Community Health, 24*(4), 291–296.

PFI (Population Foundation of India). (2014). Robbed of choice and dignity: Indian women dead after mass sterilisation. Situational assessment of sterilisation camps in Bilaspur district, Chhattisgarh. *Reproductive Health Matters, 22*(44), 91–93.

Phukan N. (2015, 3 June). *Community based monitoring on quality of care in family planning service*. COPASAH.

RamaRao, S., & Mohanam, R. (2003). The quality of family planning programs: Concepts, measurements, interventions, and effects. *Studies in Family Planning, 34*(4), 227–248.

Rattan, J., Noznesky, E., Curry, D. W., Galavotti, C., Hwang, S., & Rodriguez, M. (2016). Rapid contraceptive uptake and changing method mix with high use of long-acting reversible contraceptives in crisis-affected populations in Chad and the Democratic Republic of the Congo. *Global Health: Science and Practice, 4*(Suppl. 2), S5–S20. https://doi.org/10.9745/GHSP-D-15-00315.

References

Roy, T. K., & Verma, R. K. (1999). Women's perceptions of the quality of family welfare services in four Indian states. In M. A. Koenig & M. E. Khan (Eds.), *Improving quality of care in India's family welfare programme* (pp. 19–32). New York: Population Council.

Sangraula, M., Garbers, S., Garth, J., Shakibnia, E. B., Timmons, S., & Gold, M. A. (2017). Integrating long-acting reversible contraception services into New York City school-based health centers: Quality improvement to ensure provision of youth-friendly services. *Journal of Pediatric and Adolescent Gynecology, 30*(3), 376–382. https://doi.org/10.1016/j.jpag.2016.11.004.

Schwandt, H. M., Speizer, I. S., & Corroon, M. (2017). Contraceptive service provider imposed restrictions to contraceptive access in urban Nigeria. *BMC Health Services Research, 17*(1), 268. https://doi.org/10.1186/s12913-017-2233-0.

Scott, B., Alam, D., & Raman, S. (2011). Factors affecting acceptance of vasectomy in Uttar Pradesh: Insights from community-based, participatory qualitative research. *RESPOND Project Study Series, Contributions to global knowledge—Report No. 3*. New York: EngenderHealth/RESPOND Project.

Singh, A., Chalasani, S., Koenig, M. A., & Mahapatra, B. (2012). The consequences of unintended births for maternal and child health in India. *Population Studies, 66*(3), 223–239 (Factors influencing mistimed and unwanted pregnancies among Nepali women).

Sowmini, C. V. (1999). *A study on the self-reported reproductive morbidity in the context of contraceptive use and analysis of service determinants of reproductive morbidity* (MPH dissertation). Achutha Menon Centre for Health Sciences, Thiruvananthapuram.

Speizer, I. S., Corroon, M., Calhoun, L., Lance, P., Montana, L., Nanda, P., et al. (2014). Demand generation activities and modern contraceptive use in urban areas of four countries: A longitudinal evaluation. *Global Health: Science and Practice, 2*(4), 410–426.

Speizer, I. S., & Lance, P. (2015). Fertility desires, family planning use and pregnancy experience: Longitudinal examination of urban areas in three African countries. *BMC Pregnancy and Childbirth, 15*, 294. https://doi.org/10.1186/s12884-015-0729-3.

Stephenson, R., Bartel, D., & Rubardt, M. (2012). Constructs of power and equity and their association with contraceptive use among men and women in rural Ethiopia and Kenya. *Global Public Health, 7*(6), 618–634.

Sundari, T. K. (1999). women's experiences with the family planning program in Tamil Nadu in Improving Quality of Care in India's Family Welfare Programme:The Challenge Ahead,eds.M. A. Koenig and M.E. Khan. New York: Population Council.

Tappis, H., Kazi, A., Hameed, W., Dahar, Z., Ali, A., & Agha, S. (2015). The role of quality health services and discussion about birth spacing in postpartum contraceptive use in Sindh, Pakistan: A multilevel analysis. *PLoS ONE, 10*(10), e0139628. https://doi.org/10.1371/journal.pone.0139628.

Teshome, A., Birara, M., & Rominski, S. D. (2017). Quality of family planning counseling among women attending prenatal care at a hospital in Addis Ababa, Ethiopia. *International Journal of Gynecology & Obstetrics, 137*(2), 174–179. https://doi.org/10.1002/ijgo.12110.

Tumlinson, K., Pence, B. W., Curtis, S. L., Marshall, S. W., & Speizer, I. S. (2015). Quality of care and contraceptive use in Urban Kenya. *International Perspectives on Sexual and Reproductive Health, 41*(2), 69–79. https://doi.org/10.1363/4106915.

Vermandere, H., Galle, A., Griffin, S., de Melo, M., Machaieie, L., Van Braeckel, D., et al. (2017). The impact of facility audits, evaluation reports and incentives on motivation and supply management among family planning service providers: An interventional study in two districts in Maputo Province, Mozambique. *BMC Health Services Research, 17*(1), 313. https://doi.org/10.1186/s12913-017-2222-3.

Visaria, P., & Visaria, L. (1994) Demographic transition: accelerating fertility decline in 1980s. ECONOMIC AND POLITICAL WEEKLY. 1994 Dec 17-24; 29(51-52):3, 281–92.

Wasnik, V. R., Jawarkar, A. K., & Dhumale, D. M. (2013). Study of family planning practices with special reference to unmet need among married women in rural area of Amravati district of Maharashtra. *Indian Journal of Community Health, 25*(4), 348–353.

Yadav, D., & Dhillon, P. (2015). Assessing the impact of family planning advice on unmet need and contraceptive use among currently married women in Uttar Pradesh, India. *PLoS ONE, 10* (3), e0118584. https://doi.org/10.1371/journal.pone.0118584.

Yinger, N. V. (1998). *Unmet need for family planning: Reflecting women's perceptions.* Washington, D. C.: International Center for Research on Women.

Yore, J., Dasgupta, A., Ghule, M., Battala, M., Nair, S., Silverman, J., et al. (2016). CHARM, A gender equity and family planning intervention for men and couples in rural India: Protocol for the cluster randomized controlled trial evaluation. *Reproductive Health, 13,* 14. https://doi.org/10.1186/s12978-016-0122-3.

Chapter 6
Consensus Building on Quality of Care Priorities

Abstract We used a Delphi consensus-based approach to identify priorities for developing a research, action, and advocacy agenda for quality of care in family planning in India. The primary objective of this effort was to build a consensus among key stakeholders about research, action, and advocacy priorities to improve quality of care in family planning in India. The process included an exhaustive search using complementary approaches to identify potential research questions, and two Delphi rounds to select the priorities for developing the research, action, and advocacy agenda. This chapter presents key priorities identified through the Delphi process and qualitative inputs received from the participants. This exercise helped in soliciting inputs from a large number of individuals across diverse locations and areas of expertise. The names of participants were kept anonymous to avoid bias or domination in the process of prioritization of the quality of care agenda (research, action, and advocacy) by experts.

Keywords Research priorities · Advocacy · Action agenda

6.1 Methodology of Delphi Process

The Delphi technique is a structured process that uses a series of questionnaires or "rounds" to gather information on a specific topic. The sequence is held until group consensus is reached on the topic of interest (Boulkedid et al. 2011). We used a Delphi consensus-based approach to identify priorities for developing a research, action, and advocacy agenda for QoC in FP in India (Fig. 6.1). The process included an exhaustive search using complementary approaches to identify potential research questions, and two Delphi rounds to select the priorities for developing a research, action, and advocacy agenda.

Our search strategy included various complementary approaches to identify potential research, action, and advocacy priorities. A literature search was performed in PubMed and POPLINE, a generic search in Google, and multiple searches on the websites of government and non-governmental institutions for available

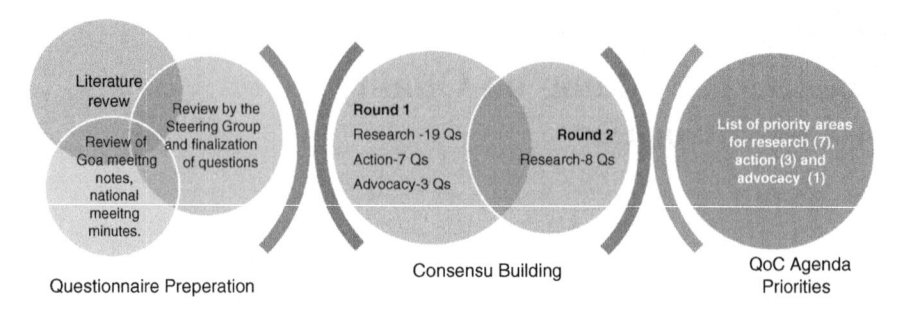

Fig. 6.1 Delphi process *Source* Authors

Diagram labels: Literature revew, Review of Goa meeitng notes, national meeitng minutes. — Review by the Steering Group and finalization of questions — Questionnaire Preperation | Round 1 Research -19 Qs, Action-7 Qs, Advocacy-3 Qs — Round 2 Research-8 Qs — Consensu Building | List of priority areas for research (7), action (3) and advocacy (1) — QoC Agenda Priorities

"grey literature". Recent studies done by ICRW and notes of the Goa meeting were reviewed. The research questions obtained from the documents retrieved in the literature search were collected and added to develop a comprehensive list of question categorized according to research, action, and advocacy priorities. This list was discussed at the first meeting of the steering group constituted under the project, held at the MoHFW on 29 November 2015. The group was asked to review the questions and suggest modifications if any.

Based on the inputs received at the steering group meeting, the questionnaire (Annexure 1), consisting of questions on the agenda for QoC in FP, was revised (19 questions on research, 7 questions on action points, and 3 questions on advocacy issues) and sent to 61 respondents representing development partners, donors, researchers, and practitioners. The selection of participants was made based on their previous knowledge, expertise, current responsibilities and engagement in FP programmes, and extensive experience of QoC issues in FP in India. The primary objective of this effort was to build a consensus among key stakeholders about the research, action, and advocacy priorities to improve QoC in FP in India. This exercise helped in soliciting inputs from a large number of individuals across diverse locations and areas of expertise. The names of participants were kept anonymous to avoid bias or domination in the process of prioritization of QoC agenda (research, action, and advocacy) by experts.

In the first round, participants were requested to participate in this iterative exercise. Questions were listed for each—the research, action, and advocacy agenda—and respondents were asked to rate their priority as high, medium, or low. We scored high as 3, medium as 2, and low as 1 to pool together views on priorities. The responses were analysed to identify top questions for furthering research on QoC in FP. We received 40% responses in the first round. The responses were analysed and ranked according to priority as high, medium, and low. Based on this, a list of questions, with high average and high standard deviation, was identified for the second round of Delphi.

During the second round, all participants were sent an email summary of the first round findings and a revised questionnaire consisting of eight questions (seven from the first round and an additional question suggested by a respondent) to the

6.1 Methodology of Delphi Process

same list of 60 people (one person opted out of the study). The second round of Delphi requested participants to rank research questions that were identified as medium priority (high average and high variance) in Round 1 and needed further analysis. The participants were requested to rank the questions as per priority on a scale of 1–8 where 1 was the highest priority and 8 the lowest. For the remaining respondents, we compared their remarks from the first round of Delphi, and found the response to be uniform. Response rate in the second round was 25%.

In both rounds of Delphi, participants also made qualitative remarks and recommendations. The summary of responses and inputs is presented in the following.

6.2 Research Agenda: Summary of Findings from First Round Delphi

Views of respondents varied from "we know what is needed so that there is very little need for research" to "we know little and much needs to be done, so most of the questions are of high priority" (Table 6.1). This section lists the questions in order of priority and presents some responses received from the respondents. Inputs related to research, action, and advocacy agendas have also been presented in Chaps. 5 and 7.

Table 6.1 Research agenda *Source* Authors

High priority	Further analysis needed		Low priority
High average–Low variance	*High average–High variance*	*Low average–Low variance*	*Low average–High variance*
• QoC metrics • Client perceptions on QoC • Factors enabling and motivating providers to provide QoC • Follow-up of clients	• Introducing additional methods • Monitoring QoC • Adolescent/youth	• Respectful care • Client–provider interaction • Financial resources • Integrating RMNCH+A *New question suggested by MoHFW* • Monitoring QoC in FP sessions	• Myths and misconceptions • Role of payments to acceptors of methods • QoC for the underserved • QoC for the urban poor • QoC to improve continuation of spacing methods • Factors determining QoC • Market segmentation • Variation in QoC

6.2.1 Research Agenda: Questions Rated as High Priority by Respondents and Key Inputs Received

1. QoC metrics: *Although we have several frameworks for QoC, a consensus about a parsimonious list of indicators perhaps has not emerged. How have studies and pilot programmes measured QoC, and what can be learnt about the use of some of these metrics at the macro level?*

   Comments: There is a need to study the relevance and utilization of QA indicators (problems faced, if any) and their impact on TFR, service uptake, and reproductive rights. We also need to understand the impact of using indicators such as TFR on measuring the success of FP. Do these indicators promote the uptake of limiting methods at the cost of spacing methods, thus adversely impacting the choice of methods? What are the other QoC frameworks being used to measure quality?

2. Client perceptions of quality: *There is some evidence that there may be divergence between the ways studies perceive QoC and the ways women (and men) perceive QoC. Clearly the interpersonal dimensions of QoC will weigh heavily with clients as they may not be able to assess the technical aspects of QoC. It would be useful to know: (a) What dimensions of QoC are important to clients? (b) What do clients perceive as their benefits from receiving QoC? (c) How important is informed choice for them? How does the social context determine the choice process? and (d) How can communities and women be engaged to ensure informed choice?*

   Comments: Understanding client (especially women's) perspectives and awareness building on client rights and components of QoC including access to services, choice, safety, privacy, confidentiality, dignity and comfort when receiving services, continuity of care, and opinion are required. This should also include standards of care and technical competency of providers.

3. Factors enabling and motivating providers to provide QoC: *Providers need a working environment that enables and motivates them to provide QoC. Although the programme has policies for a target-free approach, it is not clear how frontline staff—ANMs, PHCs—perceive this. What do providers think their benefit is in providing QoC? How has task shifting affected QoC? What factors affect providers' ability to provide QoC? How can these factors be strengthened?*

   Comments: The public sector does not have dedicated providers for FP services, so in addition to FP, the providers are responsible for several other services. Thus, enhancing their skills and empowering them with adequate infrastructure, supplies, guidance, and feedback will help in ensuring QoC. Providers' perspectives, their perceptions on how to assure quality, are equally important to understand the barriers and facilitators in providing QoC. Achievement of method-specific targets and supply-driven services may translate into focus on that specific method, thus compromising people's choice and rights.

4. Follow-up of clients: *There is a need to improve follow-up of clients. When a woman seeks clinical services for FP and is ineligible, then what options are given? How well are complications managed?*

Comments: Follow-up care, tracking and managing compliance and follow-up by service providers as per protocols is important in FP, and it is important to know where clients seek such care and how the care is provided. In addition, studies should be done to understand the reasons for discontinuation of and discontentment with services.

6.2.2 Research Agenda: Questions Rated as Medium Priority by Respondents and Key Inputs Received

1. Introducing additional methods: *Government has recently decided to introduce provision of DMPA in the public sector to expand the basket of contraceptive choices. What is the experience of DMPA introduction and what is the way forward?*

Comments: New methods should be offered within the context of choice. The impact of new methods on QoC, mCPR, and continuation also needs to be studied in both public and private sectors. Synthesis of research findings and experiences of injectable contraception delivered by NGOs would be useful to plan strategy for roll-out in the public sector.

2. Monitoring QoC: *Several recommendations have been made to monitor QoC, including community monitoring system through NGOs, monitoring by VHNSCs and RKSs, use of mHealth for direct feedback from clients, and use of HMIS with a few indictors for quality. We need to look at various experiences as to how QoC in FP is currently monitored through these mechanisms. It is not clear what the evidence is in this respect, and what more needs to be known. What research would be needed?*

Comments: The NHSRC has developed QA indicators; thus, we need to assess the relevance and usability of these indicators and monitoring mechanisms. Documentation of successful initiatives on monitoring QoC that have positively impacted the end users and have the potential for scaling up will be helpful to strengthen it further. Community monitoring of the quality of clinical services in FP alone may not be feasible.

3. Adolescent/youth: *Adolescents and young people are currently underserved and have a high unmet need for spacing methods. Government has also begun to implement the Rashtriya Kishor Swasthya Karyakram (RKSK). What would be*

needed to ensure that adolescents/young people would be adequately served by high-quality contraceptive services?

Comments: Attention needs to be paid to the preferences of youth, including unmarried adolescents/youth, and the suitability of current methods to address their unmet need. A study of demand- and supply-side strategies and enabling environment to address the SRH needs of young people will be useful. Interventions that address barriers to access quality care and improved counselling services are needed.

4. Respectful care: *How to ensure the dignity of women when they are availing of FP services? What is the current situation in this respect?*

Comments: This aspect is often found to be missing in camp settings and high-volume static facilities in the public sector. Respectful care includes not just behavioural aspects of service providers, but also the competency of service providers to deliver safe and informed choice to people. Obtaining feedback from clients about their experience of interaction with service providers will be useful.

5. Client–provider interaction: *What is the quality of client–provider interactions? How can it be improved?*

Comments: Clients' satisfaction is an important element of QoC. However, there is a need to study how these interactions help the uptake of FP services. Efforts could focus on analysing the degree and quality of interaction at various levels of service provision and reasons for no/minimal interaction. At the same time, excellent clinical procedures, without much client–provider interaction, may leave the client satisfied.

6. Financial resources: *There is evidence that measures to ensure QoC are underfunded. Some have argued that the money given as incentives should instead be used to improve QoC. There is a need to develop better estimates of the funds needed to ensure desired QoC and assess the extent of underfunding. While looking at current and needed financial resources for the FP programme, we need to also consider how well the existing financial allocations are utilized.*

Comments: It is important to study the utilization of FP funds for QoC (degree of utilization, purpose, reasons for non-utilization). Also, allocation of resources for improving and providing essential QoC instead of incentives could be explored. Often, it is the attitude of providers and current practices that determine quality.

7. Integrated RMNCH+A services: *FP is an integral part of the RMNCH+A programme. However, often FP services are not adequately integrated with other services, particularly maternal and child health services. Will better integration improve QoC for FP services? If yes, how can we ensure such integration? What should be the constellation of services?*

Comments: There is a need to study service priorities, time, and resources, etc., needed for providing integrated services. However, integrated packages for FP services may vary for clients with different needs (spacing/limiting). Counselling services are an effective entry point for providing integrated services. The IPPF has developed an integrated counselling manual to minimize missed opportunities.

6.2.3 Research Agenda: Questions Rated as Low Priority by Respondents and Key Inputs Received

1. Myths and misconceptions: *Some myths and misconceptions continue to persist, particularly on vasectomy. There is a need to look at why this is so and what can be done. Are there any successful experiences in this regard?*

   Comments: Programme strategies for involving men and developing messaging that addresses myths and increases awareness are needed. Engaging male workers, instead of ASHAs and ANMs, would be more acceptable to men. Also, provider bias against vasectomy needs to be addressed through training and supportive supervision.

2. Role of payments to acceptors of methods: *As considerable financial resources of the programme are devoted to payments (in lieu of wages foregone, etc.) to acceptors of sterilization and IUDs, there is a need to understand what role these payments play in choice and the acceptance process.*

   Comments: We need to understand the role of incentives in decision making by clients and whether it interferes with expectations of quality of service. The role of cash incentives for continuation of accepted spacing method needs to be studied.

3. Quality of care for underserved and vulnerable populations in rural areas: *Intervention research to develop cost-effective approaches to provide desired level of QoC to the underserved and vulnerable rural populations.*

   Comments: Quality care should be provided to all sections of the population. Strategies should be developed to address gaps for vulnerable populations; thus, the focus should be on the "essential level" of QoC rather than the "desired level".

4. Quality of care for the urban poor: *Intervention research to find ways to reach the urban poor with high QoC.*

   Comments: Learnings from the implementation experiences of proven strategies will be useful. Access is generally not considered part of QoC, and with most health facilities concentrated in urban areas, access and availability for the urban poor will not be difficult.

5. Quality of care to improve continuation of spacing methods: *There is some evidence that improving QoC for current users of spacing methods will improve continuation rate and reduce unmet need. Research is needed to develop effective ways to provide QoC to this group.*

Comments: There is a need to develop appropriate intervention strategies for pre-adoption of spacing methods and follow-up counselling. Review of data on discontinuation rates at different intervals, the causes, and possible solutions will help design such interventions. An option to switch over to other methods and provide improved contraceptive choices is needed.

6. Factors determining QoC: *What are the immediate factors contributing to QoC? What are the contributing factors affecting QoC? How to sustain QoC?*

Comments: A study on inputs and process in ensuring QoC would be useful to understand the key constituents of quality. In addition, a knowledge, attitude, behaviour, and practice study with service providers will be useful to develop appropriate intervention strategies. This question can be combined with behaviour change intervention for providers to deliver quality services.

7. Market segmentation: *How is the market segmented for different methods among free, mixed-subsidized, and the private commercial sector? What are its implications?*

Comments: The service delivery approaches in the public, NGO, and private sectors results in market segmentation. A study could be done with an aim to develop a balanced approach for integration of all the three sectors so that acceptance of FP can be increased.

Population Services International is currently conducting a total market approach study to better understand health markets and consumer needs by identifying market failures and determining the most appropriate interventions needed to improve demand and supply for accessible and affordable health products and services, particularly for women and girls. The overall aim of this effort is to improve market performance with a vision towards universal health coverage, which means ensuring that every person, everywhere, has access to the quality health care they need without causing undue financial hardship. The Strengthening Health Outcomes through the Private Sector or SHOPS project in India is focused on scaling up commercial health models aimed at reaching low-income consumers with essential products and services including FP.

8. Variation in QoC provided: *Quality of care may vary considerably among different implementation models. It will be useful to determine variance of different quality parameters in the different FP service delivery models, like public sector, NGO clinics, private sector accreditation sites, PPP sites, different parts of private sector, etc.*

Comments: It is important to study the variations among different implementation models to develop a comprehensive model with a common set of standards to assure QoC at all levels and settings.

6.3 Action Agenda

Table 6.2 summarizes findings from the first round of Delphi.

6.3.1 Questions Rated as High Priority by Respondents and Key Inputs Received

1. Activating QoC organizational mechanisms: *The government has devised an organizational structure for QA comprising QA officers and QACs. Several states have taken action to institute this structure. What do we know about how they function and what can be done to activate them? How do we ensure that feedback from QA assessments is shared with district officials and, if necessary, with state officials?*

   Comments: The structure and function of QACs at various levels and their impact on QoC (what elements of QoC they are monitoring) are a subject of research. It is important to examine if there is clarity of roles and responsibilities, streamlined processes, and collaborations with the concerned departments at all levels to utilize findings and recommendations of the QoC assessments in improving QoC for end users. Self-assessment methodology may be introduced to develop greater ownership and teamwork among service providers and managers.

2. Enhancing accountability of the programme. *Some have argued that the FP programme needs to become more accountable for the QoC it offers to clients and community. The programme would need to systematically assess the QoC and report the assessment results annually to all stakeholders.*

   Comments: At present, the accountability of the FP programme is vague, mostly limited to numbers and targets. A study could be done to understand what is required, where the gaps and constraints are, and how the system can be made more accountable both in quantity and in quality. Accountability also depends upon the objectives of the programme; thus, there is a need to explicitly include quality in the stated objectives. Community action and participation provide a framework for accountability of service providers through monitoring. Regular monitoring and

Table 6.2 Summary of findings from first round Delphi *Source* Authors

High priority	Low priority
High average–low Variance	*Low average–high Variance*
• Activating QoC organizational mechanisms • Enhancing accountability of the programme • Improving supply	• Periodic assessment of QoC • QoC in private sector • Strengthening role of ASHAs • Improving training

rapid surveys are already a part of the accountability framework under the NHM. However, internal mechanisms like QA, monitoring, and accreditation need to be assessed and strengthened.

3. Improving supply: *Supplies are crucial for ensuring service quality. However, some studies have reported shortfalls in the availability of supplies. There is a need to continue to strengthen supply systems to ensure availability of contraceptives down to the village level. Odisha has tested a pilot commodities logistics management system, and it is now being scaled up.*

Comments: How can the RHCLMIS implemented by the Government of Odisha be scaled up to different states in the country and the model expanded to cover the complete market? It is important to find out the underlying issues in supply chain management. What has made the Odisha model work, and can it be used in other states, if so with what modifications? Also, the model takes into account the "latest" method mix to estimate annual method-specific needs in an area. As data on method mix is not updated very frequently, and the introduction of new methods will lead to changes in the method mix, the system needs to allow for such changes. The RHCLMIS can be an integral component of the e-Aushadhi software for logistics management.

6.3.2 Questions Rated as Low Priority by Respondents and Key Inputs Received

1. Improving training: *Training of both service providers and counsellors is critical to provide QoC. The government has taken action for strengthening specific competencies. There is a need to assess and improve their competencies comprehensively. While looking at provider training, we should also consider medical and nursing education, as FP is neglected particularly in private medical colleges.*

Comments: Training alone may not be helpful in improving quality. Capacity building on the concepts, components, needs, and benefits of QoC is required both in pre-service training and subsequent induction, orientation training, and in-service training.

2. Strengthening role of ASHAs: *Government has emphasized the role of ASHAs for community-level supply of pills, condoms, and ECPs. However, some studies have reported supply shortages, lack of motivation, and inadequate training as hampering these efforts. What do we know about remedial measures that work?*

Comments: The ASHA workers are overburdened with various activities and training programmes. A study should look into the support, guidance, and regular supply of commodities available to them. Supportive supervision and streamlining health systems such as supply chain management and human resource management

6.3 Action Agenda

(training) will strengthen the role of ASHAs. Assessment of what hampers effective coordination between ASHAs, ANMs, and anganwadi workers as well as needs assessment with respect to their job satisfaction would be useful.

3. QoC in private sector: *There is a need to improve the process of accreditation and financing of private sector services to ensure the desired level of QoC in the private sector.*

Comments: Issues faced by NGOs and the private sector need to be studied in depth, particularly with respect to accreditation, empanelment, supplies, training, supportive supervision, and financing. There has been limited work on accreditation and financing of private sector services; hence, we need to determine if addressing this issue will lead to significant changes in the overall quality of FP services.

Population Services International is implementing an initiative to increase the use of LARC and long-acting permanent methods by expanding choice and access among men and women residing in the urban and peri-urban slums of 32 districts of Uttar Pradesh. Training, QA, and accreditation are key areas of focus to integrate long-acting methods provision and to encourage more consistent provider performance from existing franchises. Private sector providers are incentivized to provide these services through a more streamlined reimbursement process whereby PSI acts as the public–private interface agency.

4. Periodic assessment of QoC: *A system needs to be put in place to carry out periodic assessment of QoC that is being provided to underserved and vulnerable populations. The NHSRC has begun the process of accreditation of private hospitals for services they provide, including FP.*

Comments: The implementation of QA mechanisms is missing. Studies should look into the existing tools and reveal the constraints in implementation at the district level.

6.4 Advocacy Agenda: Key Findings of Delphi First Round

Table 6.3 summarizes the key findings of the Delphi first round with regard to the advocacy agenda.

Table 6.3 Key findings of the Delphi first round *Source* Authors

High priority	Low priority
High average–low standard deviation	*Low average–high standard deviation*
• Commitment to QoC	• Introducing additional methods • Providing additional resources for FP

6.4.1 Most Recommended Priorities and Key Inputs Received from Respondents

1. Commitment to QoC: *There is a general perception that commitment to QoC among key stakeholders needs to be strengthened. Generally, pressure for quality comes from the "voice" and "choices" available to clients and communities. How can these forces be strengthened? Are there alternative ways to increase pressure for QoC, such as dipstick studies or a system to get feedback from clients?*

Comments: Clinical standards of safe and effective provisioning and creating greater awareness of clients' rights and QoC among all stakeholders are important. Building a common understanding on QoC among service providers, programme planners and managers, policy makers, and other stakeholders is needed.

6.4.2 Questions Rated as Low Priority and Key Inputs Received from Respondents

1. Introducing additional methods: *There has been some advocacy effort to introduce additional methods. To date, the focus has been on DMPA. However, POP, LAM, and SDM may meet niche needs. Should advocacy efforts continue for their introduction?*

Comments: Advocacy for spacing methods is minimal; thus it needs to be strengthened. Method choice is very important for overall choice and for mCPR.

2. Providing additional resources for FP: *The government has pledged an additional 2 billion USD for FP 2020. Should there be advocacy to provide more financial resources to improve access, availability, and QoC of FP?*

Comments: There is need to study the utilization of available funds and advocacy for bringing transparency and accountability into the budget utilization rate. The focus should also be on expenditure and effective use of funds allocated for this year.

6.5 Research Agenda: Summary of Findings from Second Round of Delphi

In the second round of Delphi, in addition to questions rankes as 'low average and low variance' in round one, a question was added on assessing QoC in FP service delivery sessions. Respondents were asked to rank questions according to priority on a scale of 1–8 (1 = highest and 8 = lowest).

6.5 Research Agenda: Summary of Findings from Second Round of Delphi

The findings of the Delphi second round were consistent with the first round. Questions that were rated higher in the medium priority category (high average and high variance) were ranked as high priority.

1. Monitoring QoC: *Several recommendations have been made to monitor QoC, including the community monitoring system through NGOs, monitoring by VHNSCs and RKSs, use of mHealth for direct feedback from clients, and use of HMIS with a few indictors for quality. We need to look at various experiences with regard to how QoC in FP is currently monitored through these mechanisms. It is not clear what the evidence is in this respect and what more needs to be known. What research would be needed?*

   Comments: Quality continues to be a major concern in many states (ELA and reduction of fertility are still the objectives of FP services). The NHM accountability framework includes community-based monitoring and resurrecting QACs. There is a need to understand their effectiveness and impact on improving quality of services provided to clients. It could also be done by medical audits or by observing a few sampled client–provider interactions. Overall, monitoring should be supportive (or mentoring), and it should have linked incentives. Except desk monitoring through various reports, supportive supervision is minimal at the service delivery level; therefore, it is important to come up with metrics to monitor quality without making it too complicated. There is a need to ensure regularity of services and bring accountability through reinforcing monitoring mechanisms. A study is also needed on whether there is a system for acceptance of the monitoring findings, or whether that is a challenge.

2. Introducing additional methods: *Government has recently decided to introduce provision of DMPA in the public sector to expand the basket of contraceptive choices. What is the experience of DMPA introduction and what is the way forward?*

   Comments: There is a need to document system preparedness and operational processes (including staff training, logistic and supply chain management, inventory, end-point delivery, QA of product/services, follow-ups, etc.) in place for introducing the methods at service delivery points (SDPs). A systematic review of DMPA experience will inform government actions and strategies for rolling out and scaling up the initiative in the country. Qualitative primary research with clients and private providers may also be carried out. There have been concerns, particularly among certain civil society organizations (CSOs), regarding the quality of counselling and continuity in large-scale public health programmes. New methods beyond DMPA should be considered; DMPA introduction will have a very high impact and it will impact pretty much every other aspect of the FP programme (adolescent health, QoC—more methods do not equal more time for counselling, etc.), financial resources, and so on.

3. Adolescent/youth: *Adolescents and young people are currently underserved and have high unmet need for spacing methods. Government has also begun to*

implement the RKSK initiative. What would be needed to ensure that adolescents/young people are adequately served by high-quality contraceptive services?

Comments: There is need to understand the knowledge, attitudes, and practices of unmarried adolescents/youth towards contraceptive information and services, considering the stigma and cultural sensitivities attached which influence providers as well as the service seekers. A systematic review of effective FP strategies for adolescents/young people will inform RKSK. There is need to understand the current coverage of young people for contraceptive services, their fertility intentions, and the socio-cultural and service delivery–related factors affecting the use of contraceptive services by adolescents/young people. While the needs of the youth are clear through youth surveys, their preferences in terms of methods and sources of seeking methods/supplies (youth-specific market segmentation), and the differences in the needs/choices of married and unmarried youth, etc., are not clear.

4. Monitor QoC in FP sessions

Comments: Monitoring of QoC in FP services, including counselling through research and exit interviews post-FP sessions, will inform follow-up actions for improving services; this is related to client–provider interactions. For QoC, it is important to assure clients' satisfaction and acceptance of FP methods. This can be combined with monitoring QoC—comprehensive systems to monitor QoC in FP—in camps, or through individual clients at counselling centres, or even clients using products from pharmacies. Can the mechanisms being suggested there (primarily community-led) be used in service delivery sessions? Even the term "service delivery sessions" seems to refer to sterilization services only, whether in fixed-day services or in camps. Hence, this can perhaps be merged with the question on monitoring quality.

6.6 Conclusion

The present Delphi consensus identified a set of core priorities that are useful for developing a QoC agenda for research, action, and advocacy in FP in India. Suggestions were made to combine client–provider interactions with respectful care and for monitoring QoC by monitoring FP sessions.

Reference

Boulkedid, R., Abdoul, H., Loustau, M., Sibony, O., & Alberti, C. (2011). Using and reporting the Delphi method for selecting healthcare quality indicators: A systematic review. *PLoS ONE, 6*(6), e20476. https://doi.org/10.1371/journal.pone.0020476.

Chapter 7
Operationalizing the Action and Advocacy Agenda for Quality of Care

Abstract This chapter focuses on efforts to accelerate advocacy for and operationalize action on quality of care, presenting key initiatives implemented by the government and NGOs. Over the years, many recommendations have been made by researchers, activists, and observers to improve quality of care in the Indian family planning programme. These have included actions at the facility, programme, and policy levels. Many NGOs and development partners are also assisting government in implementing these measures. There is now widespread awareness and appreciation of the need to expand contraceptive choice and improve the quality of care. Quality of family planning services is a multidimensional concept, comprising various elements ranging from the provision of informed choice to adherence to standard management protocols. This chapter draws on ideas presented in various sections of this book that look at interventions, research, and commitment to addressing the unmet need for family planning in India. It dwells on the broader communication and advocacy requirements for sustaining commitment to quality of care by different stakeholders.

Keywords Accelerating advocacy · Service delivery · Guidelines
Quality assurance · Commitment to quality of care

7.1 Introduction

Over the years, many recommendations have been made by researchers, activists, and observers to improve QoC in the Indian FP programme. These have included actions at the facility, programme, and policy levels (see Chap. 1 for an illustrative list). Several actions have also been taken by the government, as mentioned earlier in Chap. 3. Under the NHM, facilities, equipment, and staffing have been improved. The fixed-day quality service approach is being implemented in many facilities. Counsellors have been appointed at high-volume facilities in some states. The government has developed guidelines and standards for service delivery. Mandated by the Supreme Court in 2005 (HRLN 2016), the government established QA structures comprising QA cells and QACs for sterilization at district and state levels. The ambit of these committees and cells was subsequently expanded to cover all RMNCH+A services. Technical guidelines for various contraceptive services have also been updated. More recently, the government has asked the NHSRC to initiate a process of accreditation of facilities for RMNCH+A services and various disease control programmes (NHSRC 2016). The NHSRC has developed assessment tools and has begun the process for district hospitals, to be extended later on to sub-district health facilities. Many NGOs and development partners are also assisting the government in implementing these measures.

7.2 The Need to Augment Action on the Ground

Quality of care has been improving. However, the improvement in QoC has been slow and needs to be accelerated. Despite investments in infrastructure, human resources, provider skills, communications, and development of guidelines and protocols, surveys and studies of the quality of FP services in Indian programmes have repeatedly shown shortfalls. Therefore, much needs to be done to improve QoC in FP services.

One of the major factors influencing the pace of improvement in QoC is the tension between achieving quantitative targets of FP acceptors and improving QoC. This pressure has reduced over time, with quantitative method acceptor targets being abandoned in 1995, but the residual effect has persisted in the form of the ELA and has replaced the earlier approach. However, having reached the replacement TFR (2.1) or lower in states with nearly 60% of the total population, and having achieved reduction in fertility elsewhere (TFR of 2.3 for the whole of India in 2014), the pressure to achieve specific performance levels has decreased. Alongside, attention to measures to improve QoC has increased, including the concern with widening the basket of choice. Nevertheless, the major advocacy objective identified by the Delphi study respondents was to increase commitment to QoC in FP services.

Reduced pressure for achieving the desired level of quantitative performance for FP acceptors has unfortunately not resulted in a corresponding increase in accountability for QoC. There are several possible reasons for this, besides the inadequate felt pressure to improve QoC. There is a measurement issue. While monitoring QoC at the facility level involves measuring several indicators, it is not clear what parsimonious set of indicators can be used at higher levels (RamaRao and Jain 2015). Second, improving QoC requires many implementation actions at the state, district, and block levels. As the capacity, commitment, and demand for improved QoC vary, state responses also differ. Third, the effort required for a culture change focused on QoC is enormous, even after enabling conditions in terms of facilities, equipment, supplies, and staffing have been met. It has taken health systems several decades to improve and reach high levels of QoC in many countries. Similar efforts around QA, QI, and systems strengthening will be needed here.

7.3 Operationalizing the Action Agenda

Three high-priority actions were identified by the Delphi study (see Chap. 6) respondents as well as by our review of interventions and research studies:

1. Activating QoC organizational mechanisms
2. Enhancing accountability of the programme
3. Improving supplies.

In what follows, we briefly discuss what would be required to operationalize these actions.

7.3.1 Activating Quality of Care Organizational Mechanisms

The government has set up an organizational mechanism for QA comprising QA cells and QACs at the district (DQAC) and state (SQAC) levels as mandated by the Supreme Court in 2005 (see Chap. 3). At that time, the major focus was on failures and complications including deaths following female sterilization. This focus continues, and the states have set up these committees. Some research shows that QoC in female sterilization services has been improving, but several gaps remain (Chap. 5). Later, the government expanded its role to cover RMNCH+A services (MoHFW 2013).

Although we do not have a definitive assessment, several commentators have observed that these committees do not seem to function well in many states. There are several barriers that constrain their effective functioning. First, the SQAC, which is supposed to monitor the functioning of DQACs, limits its work to safety issues in female sterilization. Second, often the district officials are busy with their other duties, particularly in clinical services at the district level, and may not be able to carry out field visits as needed. Third, adequate budget allotments for staffing, field travel, and other support may not be available. Finally, it is not clear what a well-functioning QoC structure can accomplish (Askew and Brady 2013).

Each of these barriers needs to be addressed. Documented experience of efforts in Maharashtra (Satia et al. 2015) suggests that a well-functioning QoC structure can help improve service quality. However, robust evidence of its effectiveness is needed to understand its potential and the actions needed to make it functional. There is a need to clarify the roles and responsibilities of QACs, their staffing, and methods of functioning, and widely communicate the same for effective implementation. There is a need to allocate adequate budgets for staffing and operations of QACs. Finally, a monitoring mechanism needs to be in place to provide supportive guidance to these committees and to solicit feedback from the findings of such committees and to communicate the same to appropriate authorities.

We now turn to a discussion of the Maharashtra experience in further detail. The Government of Maharashtra, with support from UNFPA, implemented a QA system to improve the QoC at its facilities in order to provide improved reproductive and child health services, including FP services.

A pilot project for QA was implemented in 2007–2008 in Ahmednagar district, where QA checklists were used in selected health facilities with encouraging results. Based upon a quality assessment score using the checklists, the percentage of facilities falling in "A" grade increased from 24 to 72% during the period April 2007–July 2008. The feasibility and usefulness of the intervention having been proven, the state decided to scale up the project in stages to cover all the districts. The government established a state QA cell, and a position of state QA consultant was created in the cell. District QA cells were established, followed by the creation of structures for monitoring and review. Each district constituted a DQAG under the chairpersonship of the district health officer, and consisting of 20–24 staff identified from the district hospital, the office of the district health officer, the district training team, and the hospital training team.

The intervention comprises visits by members of the DQAG to each facility once in a quarter, and using checklists identifying the actions needed to improve quality. The checklists are divided into different sections. One section collects information on the availability of trained providers, infrastructure, availability of essential protocols and job aids, equipment and instruments, availability of medicines, vaccines, contraceptives, and other supplies, and the observance of infection prevention practices. Other sections have specific questions pertaining to the programme areas of FP, maternal health and child health/immunization service provision, and performance indicators. Information on each item is collected through an interview with a service provider, observation, or looking at service records, and a score is entered against each item. Based on the total score obtained in the assessment, each facility is graded from A to D, A being very good, B good, C average, and D poor, indicating the status of RH service quality at the site. At the state level, a quarterly review meeting for QA is held under the chairpersonship of the managing director, NRHM/additional director, family welfare. The facility in-charge is accountable for implementing the action plan for improvement prepared in consultation with the DQAG. It has been observed that 60–70% of the improvements call for local action, which the facility in-charge can take using NRHM/RCH untied funds and involving the Rogi Kalyan Samiti (RKS) or patient welfare committee. District-level action is required only in 20–25% of the improvements to be made, while state-level interventions are needed to address only 10–15%.

This effort was evaluated by an independent agency in 2012. The average assessment score for the QA facilities in almost all sections of the QA checklist was significantly higher than the non-QA facilities. There was increased awareness about quality among service providers in the QA facilities compared to non-QA facilities. To varying degrees, however, almost all the districts covered under this system have succeeded in increasing the number of facilities in grade A. The QA facilities have shown better results in terms of providing privacy and confidentiality to clients, especially women, and better organization of amenities in the facilities.

7.3.2 Enhancing the Accountability of the Programme

Many have observed that the accountability of the programme for QoC is vague, and is often limited to quantitative performance. Through the Supreme Court order, QoC is narrowly perceived as safety and limited to extreme events following female sterilization. Therefore, there is a need to specify accountability "to whom", and "how".

While community and/or client feedback can be used for the four elements of the Bruce-Jain framework (Jain et al. 1992)—information provided, choice offered, continuity of care, and interpersonal relations—clients are not in a position to judge the technical quality of services provided, or the appropriate constellation of services. Trained professionals need to judge the technical aspects of services. Although the NHM used regular review missions and sometimes rapid surveys, these will not suffice for the above purpose. Therefore, QACs and QA cells were established. These are expected to assess all aspects of QoC using a variety of tools. Making them fully functional, as discussed in the previous section, will also lead to enhanced accountability.

Research is needed to enhance accountability. Periodic assessment of the QoC structure as well as dipstick studies of QoC delivered are two aspects of the research that will provide inputs to enhance accountability. However, research is also needed to design appropriate accountability mechanisms at various levels of care and service delivery. Research is further needed to identify the appropriate constellation of services and its impact on QoC.

There is also an issue of private sector accountability for QoC provided. Both social franchising and social marketing are being used widely. There are inbuilt mechanisms of accountability in both of these modes, as discussed in Chap. 4. However, it is not clear how effective they are. Also, there does not seem to be any accountability mechanism for private providers who do not fall within the ambit of these two modes.

Client feedback, as just mentioned, is a means of enhancing accountability. There are many ways in which client feedback can be sought. Very simply, clients can be asked to express their degree of satisfaction. Exit interviews have been used extensively in assessing QoC. A pilot study in Jharkhand sought to empower clients to demand QoC for maternal health using mobile technology (Gogoi and Jha 2015). It created a mobile monitor for QoC using basic mobile phones, with an interactive voice platform by which women could provide feedback on services received and, thereby, become actively engaged advocates for positive improvement of quality services. The platform also informed expecting mothers of existing health entitlements. This initiative used four QoC indicators arrived at by a consensus-building process—timeliness, service guarantee, respectful care, and cleanliness of facility—

measured by a set of 18 indicators. There was a toll-free number, which was well advertised, on which women could call and provide their rating on the QoC they received. This feedback was converted into rating scores and shared with public and private facilities to help them improve care, as well as with households to decide where to seek care. Also, women's knowledge about their entitlements improved significantly. Thus, this pilot shows the feasibility and utility of the client feedback system and can be adapted for FP, as well as scaled up.

The NHM's accountability framework includes community monitoring in addition to internal monitoring and periodic surveys and studies. Community monitoring has been proved to help empower communities in some settings. The secretariat of the group on community action is housed at PFI, which supports Community Action for Health in India. The Community Action for Health process involves strengthening VHNSCs at the village level and planning and monitoring committees at PHCs and higher levels. The programme (*a*) creates community awareness on health entitlements, and roles and responsibilities of the service providers; (*b*) collects data using a checklist to monitor health services; and (*c*) provides feedback to key stakeholders. This process has been proven to improve the overall ratings of services at the village and PHC level. It also enhances trust and improved interaction between the provider and the community, provides community-based inputs in planning and action, and reduces out-of-pocket expenditure.

7.3.3 Improving Supplies

Supplies are essential to ensure QoC of FP services, as well as to support continuity of care for users of spacing methods. While studies have identified shortfalls in supplies at the facility level for providing both clinical and non-clinical services, there is a need to continue to strengthen supply systems to ensure availability of contraceptives down to the village level.

Odisha has tested a commodities logistics management system (see Chap. 3). Learning from this experience is being used by the MoHFW to improve the logistics systems in other states. However, it is also necessary to find out how such systems can cover private and NGO service providers.

Research is needed to reveal the underlying issues in supply chain management, constraints and bottlenecks, and effective ways to manage and improve the same. It is also important to understand the entire supply chain mechanism, its gap points, and what can be done to plug these gaps.

Here we look further at how the Reproductive Health Commodities Logistics Management Information System (RHCLMIS) initiative has sought to streamline the supply chain for contraceptives in Odisha. To increase voluntary access to and utilization of FP services, the Directorate of Family Welfare, Government of Odisha, with support from UNFPA, has developed an efficient RHCLMIS to streamline administration of the contraceptive supply chain at various levels. This was aimed at guaranteeing an adequate supply of all necessary contraceptives in good condition at key service delivery points at the district, block, and sub-centre levels of the health system.

There were several challenges in ensuring availability of contraceptives and providing FP products and services to people in Odisha—inaccurate forecasting, poor tracking of supplies, and inefficient monitoring. The RHCLMIS is a multi-tier logistics management system for contraceptives, supported by a web- and SMS-based application, which helps in managing the supply of contraceptives delivered through the government at district, block, and sub-centre levels. The system deals with collection, processing, and reporting of logistics-related data at different levels, and provides instant access to contraceptive stock information and pipeline status by tracking supply and stock at all levels.

The contraceptive distribution system in Odisha needs to connect over 7000 health facilities at district, block, and sub-centre levels, and each facility needs to maintain a buffer stock of supplies to prevent stock-outs. From the state warehouse, the contraceptives are issued to intermediary levels to finally reach 6688 sub-centres manned by ANMs. The ASHAs collect the contraceptives from the sub-centres to dispense to users in the communities.

The application has various features, like instant access to pipeline stock status, data transfer through SMS, and providing alerts on stock level for indents. It is compatible with all kinds of mobile handsets. It provides automatic information on indenting with the exact quantity needed. Any level of health facility can indent between one level higher than its allotment and one level lower. The web-based portal is linked to an SMS-based system through which data on minimum and maximum stock levels is made available via SMS. Data on indents, issue, updating, and short supply is transferred through SMS. An automatic confirmation message is sent after every transaction to the sender, receiver, and supervisor. Data is transferred through the internet and via SMS to a particular short code, 56,767, with the keyword DFWO. The public has access to information on contraceptive stocks at over 7000 public health facilities in the state.

The advantage of the RHCLMIS is that it constitutes an effective management of the supply chain for contraceptives that is internet based and supported by SMS. This system provides real-time access to stock information and pipeline status at all levels. A key purpose of the RHCLMIS is to provide indication of the progress made towards the goal of increased product availability and improved logistics practices in Odisha. According to a pharmacist at a district warehouse, "Tracking supply status is easier. We haven't experienced stock-out in the past three years."

7.4 Other Actions Identified as Relatively Lower Priority

7.4.1 Improving Training

Training of both service providers and counsellors is critical to provide QoC. Government has taken action for strengthening specific competencies. Training partners like JHPIEGO, EngenderHealth, and Ipas have been working with state governments on standardizing these training processes. Research is needed to assess and find ways to improve their competencies comprehensively. While the focus has been on service providers, many programme managers also need to be oriented with regard to the concept, components, need, and benefits of QoC. Family planning is generally neglected in the curriculum of medical and nursing education, but it is not clear what can be done. Although most resources under QA are budgeted for training, one needs to keep in mind that training needs to be supplemented by facility preparedness and standard operating processes for service delivery to improve quality.

7.4.2 Strengthening the Role of ASHAs

The government has emphasized the role of ASHAs for community-level supply of pills, condoms, and ECPs. However, some studies have reported supply shortages, lack of motivation, and inadequate training hampering these efforts. Supportive supervision and streamlining health systems such as supply chain management and human resource management (training) will strengthen the role of ASHAs. Research is needed to identify the capacity of ASHAs, look at the constraints/bottlenecks in their knowledge and attitudes, as well as availability of supplies, and propose remedial measures that work through operations research. A focus on mechanisms for follow-up to ensure method continuity is essential. Tracking a couple to ensure continuous protection needs greater focus.

7.4.3 Quality of Care in the Private Sector

Increased participation of NGOs and the private sector in FP services is important. Their problems need to be studied in depth, particularly with regard to accreditation, empanelment, supplies, training, supportive supervision, and financing. The constraints and bottlenecks need to be identified and solved to get them involved in FP activities. There is a need to improve the process of accreditation and financing of private sector services to ensure the desired level of QoC in the private sector. One can build upon the experiences available on this from other areas, such as tuberculosis services.

7.4.4 Periodic Assessment of Quality of Care

A system needs to be put in place to carry out periodic assessment of QoC to identify the gaps and need for improvement, particularly for services provided to underserved and vulnerable populations. The QA cells can emphasize this aspect in their functioning.

7.5 Accelerating Advocacy for Improving Quality of Care

Over the last decade, several advocacy efforts have been made by CSOs and NGOs to reposition FP programmes in India, to expand reproductive choices, as well as to increase the knowledge of and access to underutilized contraceptive methods. The London Family Planning Summit, held in July 2012, marked a paradigm shift in the way FP programmes and services were being thought of and designed. India committed to the promotion of and expansion of access to spacing methods, and there is now widespread awareness and appreciation of the need to expand contraceptive choice and improve QoC (Satia et al. 2015).

In recent years, the government has taken several steps to improve quality by developing guidelines and standard protocols and disseminating them at national and subnational levels. The quality of FP services is a multidimensional concept, comprising various elements ranging from the provision of informed choice to adherence to standard management protocols. It also includes important features like training health service providers (in technical, clinical, and soft skills), ensuring regular supplies and services, ensuring information and counselling services that allow people to choose from a wide range of FP options, and follow-up with clients to improve method continuation rates. Government efforts are supported by several organizations that provide technical and outreach support in these areas.

This chapter draws on ideas presented in various sections of the book that look at interventions, research, and commitment aimed at addressing the unmet need for FP in India. More specifically, previous chapters have aimed to develop an understanding of the frameworks, processes, and national and some international experience of QoC. The Delphi study reinforced the need to sustain the commitment to FP, including QoC. Combined with the evidence review, it proposes research priorities for improving QoC in India. This chapter aims to discuss the broader communication and advocacy requirements for key priorities for sustaining the commitment to QoC in India by facilitation of research for improved action on the ground.

Family planning improves the health and well-being of women and families around the world. Particular attention is needed to meet the SRH needs of young people. India's response to addressing the unmet need for FP and the emphasis on a comprehensive RMNCH+A framework resonate with international efforts which are providing a platform for strengthening FP demand and services in many countries.

With a renewed emphasis on the quality of FP services, the issue is now being looked at as an essential part of a continuum of health care, and not in isolation.

There is a need to find ways to strengthen this argument and support FP programmes in the larger context of health goals within the rights discourse, and to highlight issues that concern women. Best practices and innovations, especially in India, need to be studied for replication and scale-up.

The benefits of FP are substantial. Family planning is one of the most cost-effective investments a government can make (Smith et al. 2012). Investing in FP involves several aspects which are being supported the world over. First, it is the right of every woman and man to decide the number of children and birth spacing. A continuum of care (as maternal reproductive and child health services are intertwined) is needed to help individuals and couples plan their pregnancies and to provide timely antenatal, delivery, and postpartum services. Second, because of the far-reaching health benefits, increased investment in FP and maternal and newborn health services could accelerate progress towards achieving good health for all.

India has a supportive policy environment for the FP programme. National and state policies recognize that lowered fertility rates are key to stabilizing India's population growth, so that economic and social progress can be made. Thus, policies are in place and demand for contraceptive services exists. Renewed commitment to FP will enable Indian couples to achieve their desired family size, while also reducing the impact of India's population growth on its social and economic development.

Thus, greater investments in quality FP services can help mitigate the impact of rapid population growth by helping couples achieve their desired family size and avoid unintended pregnancy and complications. The goal of this chapter is to help those working in this area to propose topics to effectively advocate for renewed emphasis on FP, and to enhance the visibility, availability, and quality of FP services for increased contraceptive use.

7.6 Past and Present Advocacy Efforts

There have been several advocacy initiatives towards improving access to FP services, some of which are described in the following subsections.

7.6.1 NGO-Led Advocacy Efforts Promoting Repositioning of Family Planning in India

Efforts led by NGOs in this arena may be categorized into two kinds:

1. *Expanding access to and choice of contraceptive methods*: This has been carried out by Advocating Reproductive Choices, a coalition of like-minded organizations supported by a rotating secretariat at PSS and the Family Planning Association of India.

2. *Repositioning FP*: This effort is spearheaded by two NGOs, the Family Planning Association of India and the PFI, pursuing the same initiative but with different emphases. The advocacy efforts have also accelerated initiatives by the government to emphasize spacing methods, expand choice through promoting NSV and IUD, improve QoC, and focus on adolescents.

7.6.2 Legal Instruments: *Devika Biswas v. Union of India & Ors (WP [C] 95/2012)*

In January 2012, a sterilization camp was conducted in Arharia district of Bihar, where 53 women were sterilized within two hours in unhygienic and cruel conditions. This camp was organized in a government school by Jai Ambe Welfare Society and authorized by the Bihar government. A petition filed in the Supreme Court highlighted the practices employed by the state to achieve sterilization targets, which were discouraged by the Supreme Court and by the National Population Policy, 2000. It also underlined how sterilization was viewed as a "population control and stabilization measure" by health care personnel, rather than as a way of safeguarding a woman's reproductive rights. The petition sought monetary compensation, directions for the safety of patients, guidelines for terms of operations, etc.

In January 2015, the Supreme Court asked the state for payments to be made to the victims under the Family Planning Indemnity Scheme. In August 2015, the Supreme Court ordered bi-monthly high-level meetings to inform state officials of the guidelines of the Government of India and the policy decisions that are modified from time to time. It also ordered state officials to implement the decisions taken at the meeting with the secretary in the MoHFW on 15 May 2015. In September 2016, the Supreme Court directed the union government to "make efforts to ensure that sterilization camps are discontinued" within three years, asking the government to persuade state governments for this purpose. The court also ordered the implementation of established legal, medical, and technical standards for sterilization. Further, it told the government to ensure proper monitoring of the programme, investigate sterilization failure, complications, or death, and increase the compensation amount in these cases. It also urged the state governments to ensure that targets for sterilization—forcing women to undergo the procedure against their will—were not fixed (HRLN 2016).

7.6.3 Social Audit as an Instrument to Improve Family Planning Services in Uttar Pradesh, 2001–2005

The Centre for Social Justice studied over 100 cases of women who had died at childbirth after the child was conceived after sterilization in Uttar Pradesh. This included women who had died during sterilization and the team had left the woman unattended and disappeared, and women who had infections/complications which were not treated in the public sector and ended up costing large sums of money. This effort verified compliance with quality standards by studying 10 sterilization camps using government-mandated quality benchmarks. The results showed that doctors were often not informed about quality parameters, did not follow infection prevention procedures or recommended surgical procedures, and women were not treated with dignity or not provided options for informed choice.

This was followed by a public hearing (*jan sunwai*)—face-to-face sharing of their testimonies by affected people—with a set of subject-matter and human rights experts, media persons, government functionaries, bureaucrats, and programme managers. This resulted in a parliamentary inquiry into the poor quality of services. Thus, advocacy based on this benchmark was successful in stopping a proposed legislation, the UP Population Control Act/Bill, and bringing the focus on quality.

7.7 What Is Needed to Advance the Advocacy Agenda for Quality of Care in Family Planning in India?

There is a need for advocacy actors and groups to rethink their agenda so as to focus on meeting the unmet needs for FP along with improving coverage and quality of services. There is a need to:

- continue the momentum around FP and promote dialogue among a broad range of national and community leaders on the health, social, and economic benefits of increasing access to quality FP services;
- working with the media to promote understanding of the benefits of FP and to increase the quantity and quality of FP coverage;
- involving men and partners to ensure an enabling environment at the community level.

India has committed to expanding access to FP for 48 million women as part of the global commitment to the FP2020 goals and as a signatory to the sustainable development goals programme. Population dynamics, reproductive and child health issues, people's access to health entitlements, and an enabling environment that protects people's right to heath are critical to sustainable development.

The government (at both central and state levels) and donor community need to invest in priority areas in research to help determine and implement the most effective and high-quality interventions for improving access to FP services. Evidence suggests that the long-term health and socio-economic benefits of increasing FP services will outweigh the costs (Kavanaugh and Anderson 2013).

Our review suggests that there is limited research available on FP and QoC in India and internationally. Although we have some evidence that FP interventions will lead to health and socio-economic benefits, more research is needed to determine how to provide and monitor quality services to create the greatest benefits for the maximum number of people.

There have been several promising interventions that have demonstrated impact in improving communication, uptake of services, QoC, and the experience of clients. These need to be scaled up with the support of strong policies and systems to put them into action.

Investing in research and action will help facilitate informed choice, increase use of FP methods, reduce unintended pregnancies, and decrease maternal and neonatal deaths and other adverse health and social consequences associated with early and closely spaced childbearing.

7.8 Key Focus Areas for Advocacy

Intervention to improve FP encompasses services, policies, information, attitudes, practices, and commodities including contraceptives that bring transformational benefits to women, men, and adolescents by empowering them to avoid unintended pregnancy and choose whether and/or when to have a child (Starbird et al. 2016). The effort to strengthen FP has to be led by central and state governments but with the active engagement of civil society, the private sector, academia, the media, and the communities.

- More investment is needed to ensure the highest level of monitoring of FP efforts. The impact of FP is long-lasting: better health, socio-economic development, and quality of life for the Indian people. By simply satisfying the unmet need and ensuring access to a broad range of methods for FP, India can increase funding for spacing methods vis-à-vis permanent methods in accordance with the unmet need for spacing methods, as part of the health budget in the states.
- Intersectoral collaboration should be fostered between the government and FOGSI to improve the quality of FP services.
- There is need to advocate for the inclusion of implants in the national FP programme.
- There is need to reactivate QA in priority states which will provide planning, implementation, and monitoring support to the FP programme.
- Availability and accessibility of FP services for adolescents should be increased through dialogue with different departments and identification of multiple entry points (education, work, sports, or other social activities) and settings (home, community, workplace, school, or clinic).
- Social mobilization should be undertaken to increase the age of marriage and raise awareness on delaying the first birth.
- Service delivery of FP products should be expanded through innovative partnerships with the private sector and civil society.

References

Askew, I., & Brady, M. (2013). *Reviewing the evidence and identifying gaps in family planning research: The unfinished agenda to meet FP2020 goals.* Background document for the Family Planning Research Donor Meeting, Washington, D.C., December 3–4.

Gogoi, A., & Jha, D. (2015). *Empowering clients to demand QoC for maternal health using mobile technology: A pilot study in Jharkhand.* In International Conference on Family Planning, Panel 199.

HRLN (Human Rights Law Network). (2016). *Devika Biswas v. Union of India & Ors* (WP [C] 95/2012). http://www.hrln.org/hrln/images/stories/pdf/Devika-Directions-Sought-May2014.pdf. Accessed February 1, 2018.

Jain, A., Bruce, J., & Mensch, B. (1992). Setting standards of quality in family planning programs. *Studies in Family Planning, 23*(6 Pt 1), 392–395.

Kavanaugh, M. L., & Anderson, R. M. (2013). *Contraception and beyond: The health benefits of services provided at family planning centres.* New York: Guttmacher Institute. http://www.guttmacher.org/pubs/health-benefits.pdf. Accessed February 1, 2018.

MoHFW, (2013). A strategic Approach to RMNCH+A. Ministry of Health and Family Welfare, Government of India.

Nadia Diamond-Smith, Martha Campbell & Seema Madan. (2012). Misinformation and fear of side-effects of family planning, Culture, Health & Sexuality, 14:4, 421–433, 10.1080/13691058.2012.664659

NSHRC, (2016). *National quality assurance standards for public health facilities.* New Delhi: Ministry of Health and Family Welfare, Government of India. (National Health Systems Resource Centre).

RamaRao, S., & Jain, A. K. (2015). Aligning goals, intents, and performance indicators in family planning service delivery. *Studies in Family Planning, 46*(1), 97–104.

Satia, J., Chauhan, K., Bhattacharya, A., & Mishra, N. (2015). *Innovations in family planning: Case studies from India.* New Delhi: SAGE Publications.

Starbird, E., Norton, M., & Marcus, R. (2016). Investing in family planning: Key to achieving the sustainable development goals. *Global Health: Science and Practice, 4*(2), 191–210.

Chapter 8
Developing a Research Agenda for Accelerating Progress on Improving Quality of Care

Abstract This chapter presents emerging priorities for research to accelerate progress on improving quality of care in family planning in India. The emerging research agenda based on our review is as follows. Client related: client perceptions of quality of care being provided in terms of dimensions of quality of care; influence of agency and autonomy of clients as well as social context and informed choice; and improving quality of care in adolescent/youth family planning services. Provider related: enabling and motivating providers to provide quality of care; effect of health system, operations, and context influencing quality of care in family planning. Programme related: quality of care improvement systems and activating organizational mechanisms to improve quality of care; quality of care metrics, monitoring system; ensuring quality of care while introducing additional methods; enhancing accountability of the programme with regard to quality of care; and benefits of improved quality of care.

Keywords Agency · Accountability · Social context · Metrics
Monitoring system

8.1 Need to Accelerate Improvements in Quality of Care

The government at the national and subnational levels and development partners including NGOs have taken several steps to improve quality of service and care in FP (Chaps. 3 and 4). However, despite these efforts, the review of available research studies shows that the pace of improvements in QoC has been very gradual and much remains to be done (Chap. 5). It has also led to the identification of research questions that need further attention. The Delphi study that aimed to pool collective views on key research, action, and advocacy agendas for improving QoC has identified several issues for improving QoC.

In view of the importance of improving QoC in increasing contraceptive prevalence and reducing unmet need so as to realize India-adapted FP2020 goals (MoHFW 2014a), there is a need to accelerate progress in improving QoC.

Based upon our analysis of QoC frameworks in FP and health (Chap. 2), we have identified potential variables to be influenced to improve QoC as those having immediate, proximate, and distal impact, direct and indirect. Direct immediate variables include competencies of providers (training, mentoring), facility, staffing, supplies, equipment, counselling materials, job aides, supportive supervision, as well as information provided to clients. The variables having immediate indirect impact include QA and QI systems, programme support systems (budgeting, planning, monitoring, etc.), and seeking client feedback on QoC received. The proximate variables having direct influence include provider targets/work expectations as well as their motivation and attitudes, incentives to users, incentives to facilitators, incentives/disincentives to providers and programme officials, as well as integration of services. In addition, proximate variables having indirect influence are those related to the health system, including the voice and participation of clients, choices available to clients, responsiveness of institutions (access, availability, acceptability, and affordability), effectiveness, and efficiency. Direct distal influences on QoC include the environment of providers (values and norms), the environment for clients (agency and autonomy, community values and norms). The political, legal, and organizational contexts of the health system (strategic vision, transparency and accountability, intelligence and information, ethics) have distal indirect influence on QoC.

8.2 What Has Been Done to Improve Quality of Care?

Our review shows that most interventions have been in the category of direct interventions with possible immediate impact. Some interventions have been in the category of indirect interventions with possible immediate impact. Very few interventions influence proximate variables to improve QoC. However, hardly any intervention influences distal variables to improve QoC.

Thus, the interventions to improve QoC have, by and large, limited themselves to making a direct impact. Perhaps there is a need to look at QoC in the broader framework of the whole ecosystem so that these interventions are seen as an integral part of the overall health system. Similarly, there is a need to empower women and communities to demand QoC when they receive FP services. This raises research questions in terms of the potential of these interventions to improve QoC in FP as well as the feasibility of influencing these variables.

8.3 Review of Research Studies

We found that the literature published in peer-reviewed journals on interventions to improve QoC is particularly sparse. Much more research is needed to identify what mix of interventions can remedy poor QoC.

We had classified research studies as those addressing the status of QoC, interventions to improve QoC, factors affecting QoC, and impact of improved QoC. A majority of the research studies on QoC refer to female sterilization services, which are progressively improving, but much remains to be done. There is very little information on QoC for other methods.

Several factors affect QoC in FP. However, our understanding of the effect of these factors remains rather limited. Provider values and norms as direct proximate variables and access to facilities as an indirect proximate variable are found to have some influence on QoC. Distal variables having a direct effect on QoC that have been studied include the agency and autonomy of clients as well as community values and norms. We need to have a deeper understanding of the effect of the health system and social environment in which providers function, as well as of the political, legal, and organizational context of the health system on QoC in FP.

Improved QoC reduces unmet need through increased acceptance and improved service utilization for contraception as well as reduced discontinuation of contraceptive use. Poor QoC may be suggestive of higher reproductive morbidity of contraceptive users. The adverse effect of unplanned pregnancy on the mother's and child's health due to unmet need for FP remains understudied and not well appreciated.

8.4 Findings of the Delphi Study

The Delphi study led to the identification of the following priority areas:

1. QoC metrics and monitoring systems
2. Client perceptions of QoC
3. Factors enabling and motivating providers to provide QoC
4. Follow-up with clients
5. Monitoring QoC
6. Ensuring QoC while introducing additional methods
7. Improving QoC in adolescent/youth FP services
8. Monitoring QoC in FP sessions.

To operationalize the action agenda, the three priority actions from the Delphi study are needed, including: activating QoC organizational mechanisms; enhancing the accountability of the programme; and improving supply. These require research support, as identified in Chap. 6. The major advocacy objective derived from the Delphi study—that of creating processes to strengthen the commitment to QoC among key stakeholders—requires an evidence base in terms of the benefits of improved QoC as well as the consequences of poor QoC, including for the unmet need for FP.

8.5 Emerging Research Agenda

We combine the three sources—actions taken to improve QoC and the gaps therein, the review of research studies, and the Delphi study—to identify a list of potential research areas (Fig. 8.1). These include: clients and their agency as well as social context; factors enabling and motivating providers to provide QoC, including their health system context; ways to measure, monitor, and improve QoC; and special issues in addressing the QoC needs of service provision to adolescents/youth and introducing additional methods of contraception. Finally, since it is critical to increase the commitment of all stakeholders to QoC, the consequences of poor QoC as well as the impact of improved QoC, including on unmet need for FP, should be identified and their magnitude assessed.

These potential research areas are classified under four themes: the status of QoC being provided, interventions to improve QoC, factors affecting QoC, and impact of improved QoC (Table 8.1). We then regroup the list of research issues as addressing the client, provider, and programme domains.

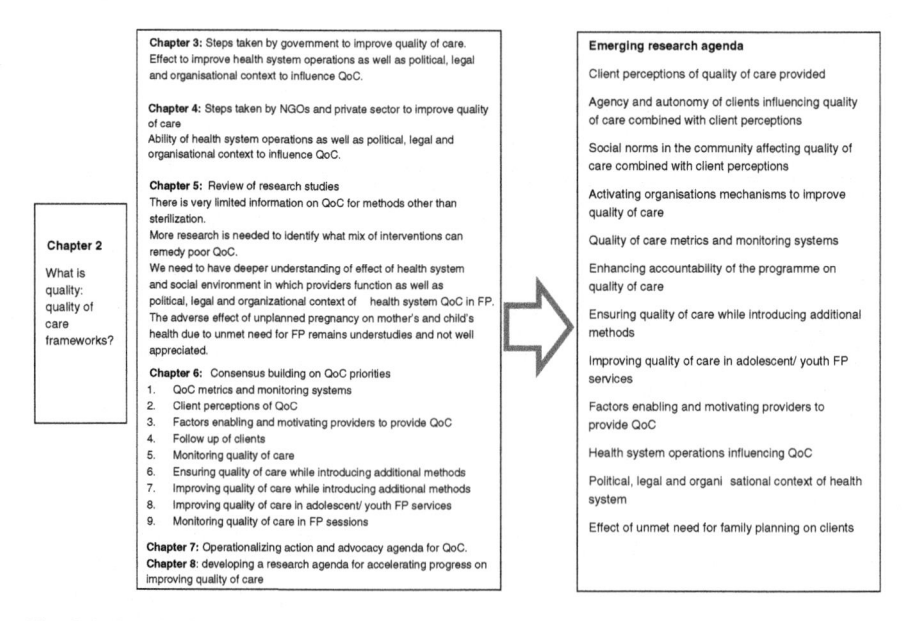

Fig. 8.1 Developing a research agenda for accelerating improvements in quality of care
Source Authors

Table 8.1 Potential research areas *Source* Authors

No.	Research area	Source/remarks	Domain
Status of QoC being provided			
1	Client perceptions of QoC being provided	Review of research, Delphi	Client
Interventions to improve QoC			
2a	QoC improvement systems	Review of research, Delphi	Programme
2b	Activating organizational mechanisms to improve QoC	Action agenda, Delphi	Programme
3a	QoC metrics and monitoring systems	Delphi	Programme
3b	Enhancing accountability of the programme with regard to QoC	Action agenda, Delphi	Programme
4a	Enhancing QoC while introducing additional methods	Delphi	Programme
5	Improving QoC in adolescent/youth FP services	Delphi	Client
Factors affecting QoC being provided			
6	Factors enabling and motivating providers to provide QoC	Review of research, Delphi	Providers
7a	Health system operations influencing QoC	Action taken to improve QoC	Providers
7b	Political, legal, and organizational context of health system	Review of research, Action taken to improve QoC	Providers
	Agency and autonomy of clients influencing QoC combined with client perceptions (area 1)	Action taken to improve QoC	Client
	Social norms in the community affecting QoC combined with client perceptions (area 1)	Action taken to improve QoC	Client
Impact			
8	Benefits of improved QoC and effect of poor QoC including effect of unmet need for FP on clients	Advocacy agenda, Delphi	Programme

8.6 Operationalizing the Research Agenda

8.6.1 Client Perceptions of the Quality of Care Being Provided

This topic covers the dimensions of QoC relating to the agency and autonomy of clients as well as social context and informed choice. Thus, the research agenda is to examine what dimensions of QoC are important to clients. What do clients perceive as their benefits from receiving high QoC?

The client-centred approach is yet to take root in the national FP programme. Thus, this area may require to be of utmost priority. Focus on the perception of quality by the end users of services is almost non-existent. Most clients are not aware of the components of QoC, their rights, choices, etc. There was general agreement by respondents of the Delphi study that the current status of client-centred QoC is poor, as can be seen from the following comments: (*a*) accordance of dignity to clients availing of FP services is no doubt poor, and is almost non-existent in camp settings and in high-volume static facilities; (*b*) rights and empowerment aspects of quality for women are completely undermined; (*c*) this is a common concern in public health facilities for women accessing care, not just for FP, and cases continue to be reported in media and in research studies. Bringing to the fore clients', especially women's, perspective on what is important and what they expect from services is critical. This will help in identifying the gaps and what needs to be done to meet clients' needs. It will make the process inclusive and bring in transparency and accountability.

Client perceptions thus need to be the focus of a primary research exercise. Several aspects of client perception need to be included:

1. *Current status of services provided*: The study should document the existing scenario at different levels and develop strategy and plans for interventions. Interventions should be delivered in a way that addresses the rights of clients. Moreover, client perception of QoC should be expanded beyond the interpersonal dimension. Clients' right to information/choice with respect to technical knowledge is also an important aspect in ensuring that they receive the essential level of QoC.
2. *Rating of services*: To improve QoC, it would be useful if clients were able to rate and comment on a public forum that is not in the control of providers or policy makers. Clients could offer feedback on: (*a*) whether they received the FP service they came for; and (*b*) whether they would recommend the provider to a family member or neighbour or friend.
3. *Respectful care and client–provider interaction*: How to ensure the dignity of women when they avail of FP services? What is the current situation in this respect? What is the quality of client–provider interactions? How can it be improved? This is particularly important for services provided to adolescents. How and to what extent do these interactions affect FP uptake and/or follow-up by clients? There is a need to find out the degree and quality of such interactions at various levels and the reasons for no/minimal interactions. This will help us understand how much effort to put into improving this element. Clients' satisfaction (an important element of QoC) is directly dependent on the client–provider interaction. However, the view has been expressed in the Delphi study as well as in some other studies that a provider who might hardly look at the patient and not talk with her, may sometimes provide excellent and safe operative care (for example, sterilization) that protects the woman or man for a lifetime. And though the service is not "respectful", the client is grateful, and it saves the woman from the risks associated with multiple births.
4. *Informed choice*: How important is informed choice for clients? How does the social context determine the choice process? How to engage communities and

8.6 Operationalizing the Research Agenda

women to ensure informed choice? Informed choice is integral to QoC. It is important to conduct awareness generation activities for the community with regard to informed choice. Informed choice is the most important aspect of counselling. It describes the process by which empowered individuals arrive at informed decisions on whether to obtain or decline treatment or services, what treatment or services to select, whether to seek and follow up on a referral, or to further consider the matter (AVSC International 1999). This would mean working on areas beyond service delivery, such as empowerment and agency for making informed choices—a process that is for and about clients.

5. *Social context*: How does the agency and autonomy of women affect their perceptions of QoC? How do community norms and values affect client perceptions? What can be done to influence social context? The community engagement component is especially weak in current efforts and in measurement. This aspect may also be studied from the provider perspective, i.e., whether providers limit the choices that they offer based on the social context of the client.

In this study, questions should also be asked of men to explore how clients (men and women) perceive QoC in the context of rights.

There are limitations to relying only on client perceptions to assess QoC. With regard to client perceptions of quality, the interpersonal dimensions weighs heavily as compared to the technical dimensions. Studies have shown that substandard services are often perceived as good-quality services, particularly by poor and underserved clients. Most findings from studies indicate that clients often rate services highly in terms of quality, even though the reality may be very different with respect to standards of care and adherence to prescribed technical protocols. For instance, the client assessment studies by ICRW (Yinger 1998) and the Population Council (Roy and Verma 1999) show that there is a wide difference between client perception and actual levels of quality of services provided in the public health facilities. There is a further need to investigate and derive a correlation between client assessment of quality and service delivery outcomes. It is therefore important that services should meet the essential quality standards.

This area can be addressed, to begin with, by survey of clients as well as qualitative research through focus group discussions. A variety of locations may have to be chosen for client surveys to cater to widely prevailing social contexts as well as QoC of services provided. Existing literature (see the studies mentioned in the previous paragraph) on the current levels of quality of client–provider interactions can help in designing this study.

As regards the *feasibility and effort required*, this is considered to be a high-priority area as indicated by several respondents of the Delphi study. Although eminently feasible, to get generalizable findings the sample size would have to be sufficiently large. The intervention research would be feasible if government, NGOs, and private sector service providers are willing to participate in this intervention research.

Its potential utility is high as: (*a*) it would increase sensitivity to client perceptions and help in assessing the current status of QoC delivered as perceived by clients; (*b*) it will lead to the identification of interventions to increase informed choice and influence social context to improve QoC; and (*c*) it could lay the basis for client monitoring of QoC provided. The interventions emanating from the study findings would aim to generate behaviour change among service providers of all categories. Such research could also result in designing beneficiary feedback mechanisms regarding providers' behaviour that will help to address this issue.

8.6.2 Improving Quality of Care in Adolescent/Youth Family Planning Services

Adolescents and young people are currently underserved and have a high unmet need for spacing methods. The government has also begun to implement the RKSK initiative (MoHFW 2014b). The question is, what would be needed to ensure that adolescents/young people would be adequately served by high-quality contraceptive services?

The category of "youth" is defined as the age group 12–25. A sizable chunk of the population consists of youth. This section of the population has different priorities which need to be addressed. The needs of married and unmarried people are different. Married couples, although covered under the programme, need education and friendly services should they wish to delay the first pregnancy or space successive pregnancies. The unmarried sexually active population has the highest unmet need, defined as: (*a*) sexually active; (*b*) wanting to prevent pregnancy; and (*c*) not using an FP method. They need non-judgemental, confidential services. The group of unmarried clients is frequently neglected. Therefore, separate studies for married and unmarried groups of clients are needed.

Possible research issues/questions include:

1. *Implementation*: The government has an adolescent and youth policy as well as a service delivery strategy. The study should look into the implementation issues, identifying the problems/constraints from multiple perspectives (such as programme managers, service providers, and clients). The implementation of RKSK in various states largely focuses on disseminating information and providing counselling services; there is no focus on improving contraceptive use among the youth.
2. *Organizing service delivery*: This aspect requires a thorough review of the "supply side", the "demand side", and "enabling environment" to address SRH needs of young people. The needs of the youth can be ascertained from the Population Council Youth study, but their preferences for access need to be studied. Also, information is needed from providers about the social contexts and biases that pose challenges (and maybe some facilitating factors). The study may also need to go beyond access to method choice—i.e., how many of the

current methods are suitable for adolescents' needs? Further, there is a need to understand barriers to the provision of quality services to this group. How can these barriers be addressed?
3. *Commercial channels*: Social marketing/commercial markets are growing for emergency contraception, condoms, and pills. There is a need to study how adolescents/youth access these channels, as there are no separate protocols for adolescents in FP. Recent policy on including contraceptives under price control would also improve use.

In this area, therefore, multiple research projects are needed. There is a need for client and provider studies utilizing mixed methods. Intervention research would also be needed to identify effective approaches in the Indian context. For this, a medium-term effort is required.

The potential utility is high, as this group has a large unmet need which may continue to increase. Success in this area will have an impact on all the components of RMNCH+A.

8.6.3 Enabling and Motivating Providers to Provide Quality of Care

Providers need a working environment that enables and motivates them to provide QoC. Although the FP programme has policies for a target-free approach, it is not clear how the frontline staff—ANM, PHCs—perceive this. What do providers think their benefit is in providing QoC? How has task shifting affected QoC? What factors affect providers' ability to provide QoC? How can these factors be strengthened?

Service providers play a very important role in ensuring QoC. Providers are the biggest barriers, or can be facilitators, in clinical FP methods (especially doctors in clinics for long-term spacing methods). This component is mostly neglected, and providers' perspectives are usually not taken into account. Provider bias is labelled as a key barrier to QoC. Research focusing on providers will help in identifying the underlying issues related to performance and in framing better strategies for improving QoC.

Provider-focused studies would explore the following research questions/issues:

1. *Perceptions of providers*: The study should reveal the perceptions of providers on QoC, its benefits, how to ensure QoC, the needs and constraints in service delivery, etc., and plan for intervention for strengthening providers' ability and motivation to provide QoC.
2. *Ways to enable/motivate providers to deliver QoC*: There is a need to study the impact of provider incentives, supervision, and improved supplies/equipment on the motivation of providers. Some observers feel that policies for a target-free approach are not fully implemented. How providers' performance is evaluated

will determine how much attention they pay to QoC. Achievement of method-specific targets will always translate into a focus on that method irrespective of clients' needs and circumstances. Research should be done on how the "target approach" can be used positively to motivate providers. This would suggest solutions that address the concerns with regard to QoC, and that can be tried and tested.

3. *Role of incentives*: The study should look specifically at the role of incentives to both providers and motivators for certain methods to see if: (*a*) it is enough to impact the choice of method that is offered to clients; (*b*) it builds the perception that FP has to be a supply-driven (push) service rather than one demanded by clients; (*c*) they will not provide/be less motivated to provide FP services if not offered incentives (this point is specifically for providers, and not motivators like ASHAs who are incentivised for each work that they do); and (*d*) whether the provision of sound incentives for spacing methods like OCPs and condoms, on the lines of those provided for sterilization, is likely to encourage providers to offer those methods too.

4. *Task shifting*: It is not clear whether there is any task shifting in FP. There are no dedicated FP providers in the system. So sometimes a provider is busy with other clinical duties, and is also called upon to provide FP services. One would like to know more regarding provider perspectives on this aspect, as FP possibly constitutes only 20% of the tasks of doctors/nurses.

5. *Providers' needs*: It is essential to address providers' needs to enable and empower them to provide high-quality services. These include the need for training, including to address gaps in providers' skills, the need for information, adequate physical and organizational infrastructure, supplies, guidance, back-up, respect from clients and managers, encouragement from supervisors, feedback concerning their performance, and freedom to express their opinion concerning the quality of services they provide. Inadequate infrastructure along with untrained support staff are major obstacles towards creating enabling environment. Therefore, research should identify how improving the quality of training, system strengthening, and accountability will improve QoC.

6. *Providers' motivation*: There is a need to use a different approach to understand "motivations", not just "efficiency" (which may be at loggerheads with quality). It may need to be addressed as a human resource issue rather than as a management problem, hence requiring organizational behaviour experts to evaluate the factors influencing providers' behaviour towards quality service provisioning. It may also include enquiring into the role of quantitative incentives in improving quality parameters.

The first stage in this research would have to be a mixed methods study to understand providers' motivations to provide QoC, barriers in their ability to provide QoC, ways to overcome these barriers, and strengthen their working environment. It could also include health system operations (the voice and participation of clients, choices available to clients, responsiveness of institutions [access, availability, acceptability, affordability], effectiveness and efficiency) influencing

QoC (research area 7a in Table 8.1). Depending upon the findings, rigorous intervention research should be designed.

As the problem is serious, this study would need to be undertaken. However, it could proceed in phases that could be further divided into sub-studies. The potential utility of such research is high if it enables better understanding of the factors affecting providers' ability to provide QoC. This in itself could lead to programme managers taking steps to strengthen their programme and improve the QoC provided.

8.6.4 Effect of Health System Operations Influencing Quality of Care in Family Planning

Health system operations have a proximate indirect influence on QoC in FP, as FP services are provided in health facilities. Even non-clinical methods provided at the community level are guided by health system operations.

Several features of health system functioning influence QoC in FP, including the voice and participation of clients, the choice available to clients, the responsiveness of institutions (access, availability, acceptability, affordability), effectiveness and efficiency. It is important to know which operations of the health system have an influence on which dimension of QoC in FP, and in what way. This would lead to possible interventions at the health system level for optimal and sustainable improvements in QoC for FP.

The following research issues/questions may be explored:

1. *Role of voice and choice*: Does strengthened voice and increased choice allow client and community feedback to influence providers and managers to improve QoC? It should be noted that this may not ensure quality in the technical dimensions of care.
2. *Adherence to protocols*: This is a general feature of health services. Actions taken to improve QoC, for instance, have shown how actions to improve clinical practices in maternal health also provide traction for the same improvements in FP. Infection control practices are also likely to affect all services.
3. *Counselling*: This aspect is of critical importance for QoC in FP, although it may not be perceived as having significant importance for other health services. Therefore, counselling may not generally be valued highly. A study of counsellors appointed by the government for FP found that their potential was not fully realized due to the operational practices of the facilities (see Chap. 4).
4. *Informed choice*: As an important dimension of QoC, informed choice requires joint decision making between the client and the provider. This is often not the case for patients seeking other curative services. Therefore, people wanting to get FP services are referred to as "clients" rather than "patients", as they are not sick.

Thus, it would be useful to assess how health system operations are facilitating/constraining improvement in particular dimensions of QoC. This will require a mixed methods study covering sites where health system operations differ and assessing both health system functioning and the QoC delivered. It is feasible provided government, NGOs, and private service providers are interested. Insights into the nature of the relationship between health system functioning and QoC would lead to more effective and sustainable QoC interventions.

8.6.5 Political, Legal, and Organizational Context of the Health System

It has been hypothesized that the political, legal, and organizational context of the health system may have distal indirect influence on QoC in FP. Although not definitive, the specific dimensions of context include strategic vision, transparency and accountability, intelligence and information, and ethics.

It is not clear how the context affects QoC in FP. For instance, a strategic vision comprising not only coverage but also quality of health services would promote QoC in FP. The sharing of evaluations of services with the community would bring pressure to bear on facilities and service providers for QA.

These relationships are not well understood. Therefore, in the first stage, it would be useful to carry out exploratory research. It is difficult to say whether concrete interventions to improve QoC in FP would emerge. Also, interventions would have to be at the health system level. Therefore, the utility of such study would be long-term. However, since our understanding of this aspect is very weak, some effort needs to be undertaken.

8.6.6 Activating Organizational Mechanisms to Improve Quality of Care

The government has devised an organizational structure for QA comprising QA officers and QACs. Several states have taken action to institute this structure. The study of QACs' structure and function is very important, as it is the mechanism that the government is relying upon to improve QoC. In most states, the system is either physically not present, or, even if it has been set up, it is non-functional.

The following research issues/questions arise in this area:

1. *Functionality*: The functioning of QACs and its impact on QoC (based on what elements of QoC they are monitoring) should be a subject of research. It will be important to learn whether these structures are functional, how effective they are, who is accountable for managing and making them effective, and whether they have the required resources, authorities, and capacities.

2. *Roles and responsibilities*: It is very important to understand the role of state and district QACs. It is important to have clarity on their roles and responsibilities and what can be done to activate them. How do we ensure that feedback from QA assessments is shared with district officials and, if necessary, with state officials?
3. *Improving effectiveness*: Identification of roles and responsibilities, streamlined processes, and collaboration with the concerned departments at all levels are needed to utilize the findings and recommendations of the QoC assessments for improving QoC for end users. Self-assessment methodology may also be introduced to develop greater ownership and teamwork among service providers and managers.
4. *Staffing*: Often, DQACs do not work well as officials in the districts have many other responsibilities, and they cannot set aside their clinical duties for QA visits. An alternative way to staff these committees needs to be explored.

It is of the utmost importance to understand the mechanisms for improving quality. This needs to be approached by observation of committees' functioning, interviews with key officials involved, and the review of documents pertaining to the committees' functioning. Such research is eminently feasible provided there is government buy-in. Since QACs are the mechanism that government is relying on to assure QoC in FP, and their mandate has been expanded to cover all RMNCH+A services, it would be useful to enhance their effectiveness. Experience shows that a modest amount of financial and human resources would be required to implement the recommendations arising from such research.

8.6.7 Quality of Care Metrics, Monitoring System, and Enhancing Accountability

8.6.7.1 Quality of Care Metrics

We have several frameworks for QoC. However, a consensus about a parsimonious list of indicators has not emerged. Quality of care is an overarching issue and it is important to come up with metrics to monitor quality without making it too complicated. The research will generate evidence and understanding for policy and programme making. It is important to build consensus on indicators for QoC at all levels—from the district to the national level. The progress and results may then be assessed against these indicators. This will ensure that policy makers, programme managers, and service providers have a common understanding about QoC indicators. Therefore, it is critical to select the right indicators, sources of data, and periodicity of reporting.

The following research issues/questions arise in this regard:

1. *Documentation*: How have studies and pilot programmes measured QoC and what can be learnt about the use of some of these metrics at the macro level? Recent work on QoC in FP2020 will be useful for this study. We can also look at whether PMA2020 and Track 20 are measuring quality, and if so, how and at what level.
2. *Developing indicators*: There is a need to look at different perspectives (those of different users, providers, managers, etc.). Quality of care metrics should start with clinical standards of care in different settings—outreach, camp, and fixed facility. There is a greater consensus on clinical quality indicators but much less on rights and empowerment indicators. There are frameworks having elements and sub-elements of QoC in FP. Indicators would follow from these frameworks. Depending on programme need, levels of care and maturity in these frameworks can be adapted. The quality frameworks provided by the Donabedian model (Donabedian 1988), the Bruce-Jain framework (Bruce 1990; Jain 1989), and WHO (WHO 2016) and UNFPA (2015) have generated programme domains and QoC indicators for measurement and monitoring, but these could not be effectively integrated/implemented in large programmes for diverse reasons: challenges in collecting, consolidating, and analysing QoC data for decision making; lack of resources and mechanisms; and even differences in defining the essential quality standards. There is a need to understand what other frameworks (apart from the Bruce-Jain and Donabedian frameworks) are being used to measure quality and to develop a comprehensive list of indicators that incorporate qualitative aspects of quality, apart from the direct service delivery statistics. Moreover, when FP is being mainstreamed with other clinic consultations, it may not be very attractive to measure just the FP indicator list.
3. *Use of indicators*: The Government of India in association with the NHSRC (2013) has developed indicators for QoC that are both facility based and for specific services, along with operational guidelines for QA in public health facilities. Research should aim to study how those indicators are utilized, problems faced if any, the relevance and utilization of those indicators, and the need to modify them for better utilization at the macro level.
4. *Impact of indicators*: Apart from indicators for measuring QoC in FP, we also need to judge the impact of using indicators such as TFR on measuring the success of FP in general, especially whether such indicators promote the uptake of limiting methods at the cost of spacing methods, thus adversely impacting the choice of methods. Also, how do we measure the reproductive rights element of FP (starting from achieving the desired family size, which is usually not covered in the frameworks)?

This could be a secondary research exercise, documenting the metrics used and the experience with their measurement and effectiveness. International experience will also help in identifying various metrics used. If this process could be used to build a consensus on quality metrics at various levels of the programme and for different stakeholders, then it would have high utility.

8.6.7.2 Monitoring Quality of Care

Several recommendations have been made to monitor QoC, including the community monitoring system through NGOs, monitoring by VHNSCs and RKSs, use of mHealth for direct feedback from clients, and use of HMIS with a few indicators for quality.

It is often said that if it cannot be measured and monitored, then it cannot be improved. Monitoring and supportive supervision, therefore, play a vital role in improving QoC. Quality of care indicators, their inputs, and processes are well laid out by Government of India documents. The problem is their implementation and monitoring. Except desk monitoring through various reports, monitoring and supportive supervision are very minimal at the service delivery level. Periodic internal quality audit could be carried out by in-house teams such as QACs, whereas external quality audit could be conducted by a third party to help monitor and assess QoC.

The following research issues/questions may be examined:

1. *Documentation*: There is a need to look at various experiences with regard to how QoC in FP is currently monitored through these mechanisms. It is not clear what the evidence is in this respect, and there is need to document what is known and what more needs to be known. What are the promising practices and mechanisms for monitoring of QoC? What research would be needed? There is also a need to study whether a system exists for the acceptance of the findings of monitoring, or whether that is a challenge because there is no point of "monitoring" unless the findings are used for improvement (closing the complete monitoring and improvement loop).

    A combination of approaches needs to be used for monitoring of QoC, as one size doesn't fit all. Many models, such as those listed here, have been tried in different states of the country. It would be useful to identify and document successful initiatives that have impacted end users positively and have the potential for scaling up. What are the methodologies and indicators of quality for the FP and SRH services in these initiatives?

2. *Monitoring process*: The Government of India in association with the NHSRC has developed detailed monitoring indicators, and minimal, basic indicators have also been culled out for QA in FP services. The study should look into those indicators for their relevance and user-friendliness for various FP services, as also existing monitoring mechanisms, like who does what, at what frequency, what is the outcome, how the findings are utilized, etc.

3. *Approaches to monitor QoC*: There is a need to monitor the QoC of different components. This could be done by medical audits or by observing a few sample client–provider interactions. Helplines have also been used for client satisfaction

surveys to monitor quality. The monitoring of QoC in FP services, including counselling, through research and exit interviews post-sessions will inform follow-up actions for improving the effectiveness of services. There is a need to look at comprehensive systems to monitor QoC in FP as part of any service delivery system, be it individual clients at counselling centres or even clients using products from pharmacies. Overall monitoring should be supportive (or mentoring) and should have linked incentives.
4. *Community monitoring*: Views on community monitoring vary. One view is that we should identify other ways to monitor quality, especially community-led monitoring. There is monitoring of QoC through Community Action for Health, which provides a framework for accountability of service providers through community participation. This framework has been used in several states (for example, Maharashtra and Bihar). mHealth interactive voice response system (IVRS) has also been used for community monitoring of health indicators, including QoC. One of the challenges cited in such studies is that it becomes difficult to segregate the FP experience from the broad array of health services monitored through community-based monitoring. Research is needed to generate evidence on results from these and many other innovative initiatives/pilots, and the scalability potential thereof.
5. *Monitoring technical quality of services*: A contrary view is that community monitoring of the quality of clinical services is a myth. How would the community know if proper asepsis was maintained during surgery or analgesia/sedation was adequate? The hospital management information system, on the other hand, provides information on complications and failures of sterilization. How could community monitoring have prevented the Bilaspur sterilization deaths? Therefore, internal QA/monitoring/accountability/accreditation mechanisms need to be assessed and strengthened.

Research in this area could begin with documentation of various monitoring systems used, their operation, and their effectiveness. This would need to be followed up by evaluating possible options for a monitoring system emerging out of the documentation. Overall, this would be a medium-term effort. If the government, NGOs, and private service providers use the monitoring system thus developed, then this research would be of high utility.

8.6.7.3 Enhancing the Accountability of the Programme

Some have argued that the FP programme needs to become more accountable with regard to the QoC it offers to clients and communities. The programme would need to assess QoC systematically and report the assessment results annually to all stakeholders.

Accountability depends upon the objective of the programme. The programme may first need to explicitly include quality in its stated objectives. At present, the accountability of the FP programme is very vague, mostly limited to numbers, i.e., achieving targets; none exists for QoC. Currently the focus on activities for promoting quality in FP services is diluted by the focus on increasing the canvas and scope of QA mechanisms.

Quality continues to be a major concern in many states, where achieving ELA and reduction of fertility are still the objectives of FP services. While it may be argued that overall quality enhancement will improve FP acceptance and prevalence, in reality it may not, when sterilization and IUCD performance continue to be reviewed in terms of achieving ELA. There is a need to ensure regularity of services and bring in accountability for quality through reinforcing monitoring mechanisms.

This research is related to the areas of quality metrics and monitoring systems discussed earlier. The NHM has an accountability framework, which includes community-based monitoring and resurrecting QACs. Mostly, the programme does not have formal mechanisms for accountability to the community. Hence the need to understand their effectiveness and impact on improving quality of services provided to clients. Internal audits, regular monitoring, and rapid surveys are already a part of the accountability framework under NHM. This study should highlight what is required, identify where the gap is, what the constraints are, and how the system can handle proper accountability both for quantity and quality. There is also a need to specify how to report and at what forums and periodicity.

Accountability would build on the monitoring systems for QoC that are currently used or will be developed. More immediately, client perceptions and observations of adherence to technical protocols either through external audits or through QA mechanisms might enhance accountability in the short term. These would have to be refined for use. This research is feasible provided there is pressure on the system for enhanced accountability. If accountability for delivering QoC is enhanced in both district- and national-level programmes, then a large number of current users would benefit. It may also contribute to reducing the unmet need for FP.

8.6.8 Ensuring Quality of Care While Introducing Additional Methods

The government has recently decided to introduce the provision of DMPA in the public sector to expand the basket of contraceptive choices. What has been the experience of DMPA introduction, and what is the way forward to ensure QoC while introducing additional methods?

Quality of care is critical while introducing DMPA to ensure continuation of use. Counselling, use experience, and knowledge of where to seek help are important. Further, follow-up with clients is needed to ensure continuity of care. For instance, providing a helpline as part of a private introduction of DMPA reduced the discontinuation rate. Providing the requisite QoC will be needed for successful introduction of DMPA. It will also provide experience, as other methods will be introduced in the programme.

Research issues/questions in this area might include:

1. *Documentation*: There is considerable experience in the NGO and private sector as well as in neighbouring countries such as Nepal and Bangladesh, and studies are available (Population Council and Dimpa evaluation). Further, DMPA was also introduced in the public health system in Rajsamand district as a pilot project. So a synthesis of research findings and experiences on the delivery of injectable contraception by NGOs as well as the public sector will be useful for the introduction of injectable contraception in public health sector (Khan et al. 2015).
2. *Study focus*: The study will need to focus on the knowledge and perceptions of both providers and clients, as it is being introduced in the public sector. Effective counselling needs to be made an integral part of the programme to dispel myths and misconceptions and to deal with common side effects. Two issues from the QoC perspective are: Is the method offered within the context of choice? And what is the impact of expanded choice on QoC, continuation of contraceptive use, and prevalence rate?

As DMPA is being introduced by the government and resources are expended in introducing it, it would be feasible to conduct these studies as implementation research. This research will help in institutionalizing DMPA service delivery with appropriate QoC and promote full realization of the benefits of DMPA introduction. Since this might become a reference point for introducing other, newer methods, there is a need to document the DMPA roll-out from the system's planning perspective.

8.6.9 Benefits of Improved Quality of Care

There is a general perception that commitment to QoC among key stakeholders needs to be strengthened. Perhaps there is insufficient understanding of the consequences that clients face when they receive inadequate QoC, including the consequences arising from unmet need for FP (unwanted or mistimed pregnancies and the consequences thereof).

To prioritize improvement and to sustain quality, therefore, it is essential that commitment of various stakeholders is built and maintained. Generally, FP administrators prioritize improving access over improving the quality of current services, as long as these services are seen to be improving contraceptive prevalence. Some measures such as adding new methods to the programme also improve prevalence. Improving access is also justified as increasing equity. However, the trade-off between improving access and quality shifts as near-universal access and a high level of coverage is achieved. This point of inflection is not always clear unless improving access does not improve coverage significantly, or improved coverage

8.6 Operationalizing the Research Agenda

does not result in corresponding improvement in prevalence. Therefore, evidence-based advocacy is necessary for increasing priority for QoC.

To support advocacy for prioritization of improving QoC, it is necessary that benefits of improved QoC are comprehensively studied. There is evidence that improved QoC increases facility utilization and reduces unmet need for FP. It not only reduces side effects or complications arising out of contraception, but also reduces their adverse impact on health. The clients experience overall improved service experience and contraceptive use. Poor QoC produces the reverse effects. Studies on the impact of improving QoC have focused on one or more of the above effects, but have not comprehensively studied them.

The adverse consequences of too many, too close, and too early pregnancies are also widely known. However, the consequences of unwanted pregnancies (abortions, impact on maternal and child health) and mistimed pregnancies (suboptimal birth intervals, impact on maternal and child health) are underappreciated.

Research issues/questions in this area may include the following:

1. *Impact*: It would be useful to relate improvements in QoC to facility utilization, reduced quantum and severity of side effects or complications arising from contraceptive use, reduced unmet need, reductions in unwanted and mistimed pregnancies and their adverse impact on maternal and child health, and overall client experience.
2. *Perceptions of stakeholders on QoC*: An in-depth study on this issue is important to find out the perception/views of programme managers and clients/communities on the benefits of improved QoC as well as of the consequences of poor QoC.
3. *Increasing commitment to QoC*: What are the ways to increase pressure for QoC, such as dipstick studies or a system to get feedback from clients?

It would be useful to undertake mixed method studies in comparable areas with differing QoC. Cohort or panel studies are not common in FP. Therefore, prospective or recall studies may need to be utilized to understand the impact of unmet need. Based on available data, perhaps modelling can be undertaken for this propose. This may require a modest effort. It may be useful for sustaining commitment to QoC among clients/communities, programme managers, and service providers.

8.7 Summary and Conclusion

Realizing India's FP 2020 goals requires significant reduction in the unmet need for FP. Women/couples with unmet need do not practise contraception for three main reasons: (*a*) they do not feel at risk of becoming pregnant; (*b*) they are opposed to the use of contraception; or (*c*) they fear side effects and health risks. While communication strategies to change individual and community norms are needed to reduce opposition, QoC needs to be improved to address the fear of side effects and health risks. Research evidence shows that providing the right information at the right time, expanded contraceptive choice, and improved client–provider interaction can increase contraceptive prevalence and facility utilization as well as reducing the discontinuation of contraceptive use (see Chap. 5). In view of the predominance of sterilization in India's contraceptive method mix, discontinuation has not received much attention in India. However, it is likely to gain importance as spacing method use increases. There is a need to conduct research on priority areas. Table 8.2 summarizes the nine areas of research that have emerged from a synthesis of available literature, experiences from interventions, and Delphi findings.

To realize FP2020 goals, the focus has been on increasing the capacity to deliver contraceptive services by training providers, including for offering PPIUCD, increasing the reach of social franchising, expanding the availability of methods by including DMPA, POP, and Saheli (weekly pill) in the public programmes, and launching a new communication campaign emphasizing the beneficial effect of contraceptive use on the mother's and child's health.

Many measures have also been taken by the government to improve QoC in FP including improving facilities, providing equipment, appointing counsellors at high-volume facilities, establishing a mechanism for QA through QA cells and committees at district and state levels, as well as initiating an accreditation process for health facilities (Chap. 3). While QoC has improved, progress in improving QoC has been slow as recent studies indicate, particularly in providing informed choice and adhering to technical protocols (Chap. 5).

Evidence-based interventions to accelerate improvements in QoC need to be implemented through an appropriate research agenda to enhance progress towards realizing FP 2020 goals. This background paper has laid out an agenda for this purpose.

8.7 Summary and Conclusion

Table 8.2 Summary of types of research and potential utility of each research area
Source Authors

No.	Research area	Type of research	Potential utility
1	Client perceptions of the QoC being provided in terms of dimensions of QoC, influence of agency and autonomy of clients as well as the social context, and informed choice	Survey of clients and qualitative research in several locations	Increased sensitivity to client perceptions and assessment of current status of QoC delivered as perceived by clients; identification of interventions to increase informed choice and influence the social context to improve QoC; and providing a basis for client monitoring of QoC provided
2	Improving QoC in adolescent/youth FP services	In this area, multiple research studies are needed. There is need for client and provider studies utilizing mixed methods. Intervention research would also be needed to identify effective approaches in the Indian context	The potential utility of such research is high as this group has a large unmet need which may continue to increase. Success in this area will have an impact on all the components of RMNCH+A
3	Enabling and motivating providers to provide QoC	Mixed methods study to understand providers' motivations, identify barriers and ways to overcome these barriers, and strengthen their working environment; health system operations; rigorous intervention research	Programme managers taking steps to strengthen their programme and improve QoC
4	Effect of health system operations influencing QoC in FP	Mixed method study covering sites where health system operations differ and assessing both health system functioning and QoC delivered	Increased effectiveness of interventions to improve QoC
5	Political, legal, and organizational context of health system affecting FP	Exploratory research	Long-term utility in improving QoC
6	QoC improvement systems and activating organizational mechanisms to improve QoC	Observation of committees' functioning, interviews with key officials involved, and review of documents pertaining to committees' functioning	Potentially enhanced effectiveness of QA mechanism

(continued)

Table 8.2 (continued)

No.	Research area	Type of research	Potential utility
7	QoC metrics	Secondary research	Building consensus on metrics to be used at various levels
	QoC monitoring system	Documentation of various monitoring systems used, their operation, and effectiveness. Evaluation of possible options for monitoring	Use of agreed-upon monitoring system would have high utility for improving QoC
	Enhancing accountability of the programme with regard to QoC	Building on the monitoring system for QoC in 7b above, including client perceptions and observation of adherence to technical protocols	A large number of current users would benefit. Reducing unmet need
8	Ensuring QoC while introducing additional methods	This would be implementation research, as DMPA is currently being introduced	This research will help in institutionalizing DMPA service delivery with appropriate QoC and promote full realization of the benefits of DMPA introduction. Since this might become a reference point for introducing other newer methods, there is a need to document the DMPA roll-out from the system's planning perspective
9	Benefits of improved QoC and consequences of poor QoC including impact of unmet need for FP on clients	Comparison of areas with varying QoC. Analysis of available retrospective and prospective data, modelling research	Evidence-based advocacy for enhancing and sustaining commitment to QoC

References

AVSC International. (1999). *Self-assessment for supervisors and managers.* New York: AVSC International.

Bruce, J. (1990). Fundamental elements of the quality of care: A simple framework. *Studies in Family Planning, 21*(2), 61–91.

Donabedian, A. (1988). The quality of care: How can it be assessed? *Journal of the American Medical Association, 121*(11), 1145–1150. https://doi.org/10.1001/jama.1988.03410120089033.

Jain, A. K. (1989). Fertility reduction and the quality of family planning services. *Studies in Family Planning, 20*(1), 1–16.

References

Khan, M. E., Dixit, A., Ahmad, J., & Pillai, G. (2015). *Introduction of DMPA in public health facilities of Uttar Pradesh and Rajasthan: An evaluation*. New Delhi: Project Brief, Population Council.

MoHFW (Ministry of Health and Family Welfare). (2014a). *India's vision FP2020*. New Delhi: Family Planning Division, Government of India.

MoHFW (Ministry of Health and Family Welfare). (2014b). *Strategic guidelines*. Rashtriya Kishori Swasthya Karyakram.

NHSRC (National Health Systems Resource Centre). (2013). *Operational guidelines for quality assurance in public health facilities*. New Delhi: Ministry of Health and Family Welfare, Government of India.

PMA2020. https://pma2020.org/research/country-reports/india. Accessed July 26, 2017.

Roy, T. K., & Verma, R. K. (1999). Women's perceptions of the quality of family welfare services in four Indian states. In M. A. Koenig & M. E. Khan (Eds.), *Improving quality of care in India's family welfare programme* (pp. 19–32). New York: Population Council.

TRACK20. http://www.track20.org/pages/countries_country_page.php?code=IN. Accessed July 26, 2017.

WHO (World Health Organization). (2016). *Quality of care in contraceptive information and services, based on human rights standards: A checklist for health care providers*. Geneva: World Health Organization.

WHO (World Health Organization), & UNFPA (United Nations Population Fund). (2015). *Ensuring human rights in contraceptive service delivery: Implementation guide*. Geneva: WHO, New York: UNFPA.

Yinger, N. V. (1998). *Unmet need for family planning: Reflecting women's perceptions*. Washington, D.C.: International Center for Research on Women.

Chapter 9
Enhancing Demand for Quality of Care in Family Planning in India: A Consultation Report

Abstract In this final chapter, we present a summary of a consultation held in January 2017 on enhancing demand for quality of care in family planning in India. All available evidence indicates that quality of care in family planning is only improving gradually. Compared to interventions and research to increase the capacity of the service delivery system to provide quality of care, there are very few interventions that focus on enhancing demand for quality. Issues affecting quality of care extend beyond the service provider setting, influencing clients before they arrive to seek services. Important determinants that affect the demand for quality of care include clients' agency and autonomy, gender norms, socio-cultural factors, costs of seeking quality care, myths and misconceptions about methods, and access to services and products. Clients' perspectives on the services they receive are an essential part of understanding and assessing quality of care, and these are shaped by cultural values and norms, past experiences, perceptions of the role of the health system, and interactions with providers. There are several opportunities for improving quality of care. Socio-economic status, particularly of women, is gradually improving. The information and communication revolution offers opportunities to empower clients and communities to enhance demand for quality of care. The trade-off between increasing access and improving quality is shifting in favour of quality.

Keywords Gender · Social norms · Costs of seeking quality care
Client perspectives

9.1 Why Focus on Enhancing Demand for Quality of Care?

This chapter presents a summary of deliberations held at a two-day consultation titled "'Quality Refresh': Taking Stock and Exploring New Pathways to Enhancing Demand for Quality of Care in Family Planning in India—Developing Our Research and Advocacy Agenda" held on 16–17 January 2017 in Jodhpur, Rajasthan (Satia and Chauhan 2017). This consultation brought together more than

40 participants (representatives of donor organizations, researchers, programme planners, policy analysts, and health activists). The agenda of this meeting was to further the ongoing discussion on QoC in FP and to contribute new ideas to build the discourse around this important issue in India. In addition, it was proposed that the learnings from this meeting would have practical value to the participants in charting the future of QoC research and advocacy in their respective organizations.

Access to quality services can be achieved if women are cared for in their own communities by service providers, and are empowered to take decisions about their own health in a supportive environment. This can be made possible by supportive demand-side interventions at the community and health systems levels, and by bringing about a positive shift in social norms that give importance to women's right to health. Available literature and experiences from the field focus more on direct, service delivery interventions for improving QoC (see Chaps. 3, 4, and 5). Therefore, there is a need to develop strategies and research that focus on enhancing demand for QoC.

9.2 What Does the Available Evidence Indicate?

All available evidence indicates that QoC is only improving gradually. Compared to interventions and research to increase the capacity of the service delivery system to provide QoC, there are very few interventions that focus on enhancing demand for quality (Table 9.1 and Annexure 2). Our review of research on and interventions to improve QoC is presented in Table 9.1.

There are several opportunities for improving QoC. For example, socio-economic status, particularly of women, is gradually improving. With advancements in information and communication technologies, there are far greater opportunities and mediums available to empower clients and communities to spread awareness and enhance demand for QoC. The trade-off between increasing access to services versus improving QoC is shifting in favour of quality.

During the Jodhpur consultation, participants' perspectives on enhancing demand for QoC in FP clustered around nine interrelated themes which includes the following:

1. Clients at the centre of QoC
2. Empowering young people to demand QoC
3. Engaging the community
4. Working with other sectors
5. Communication for enhancing demand
6. Governance
7. Accountability
8. Advocacy
9. Service provision.

9.2 What Does the Available Evidence Indicate?

Table 9.1 Interventions for enhancing demand for quality of care in family planning

Intervention focus	Examples
Client education and message reinforcement	– Helpline: Dimpa, Saadhan—PSI – Complementing helpline service with FAQ: Pahel, PSI – Use of mHealth platform to assist clients for informed choice – QoC as a part of FP demand generation communication: research – Comprehensive campaign: integrated FP services
Client feedback	– Empowering clients to demand QoC using mobile technology: Centre for Catalyzing Change (C3) – Improving management: including patient feedback: Karuna Trust – Follow-up mechanism for client feedback: Ipas – Client satisfaction surveys: Ujjwal Project
Enhancing gender equity	– Education of couples and expanding the role of husbands: CHARM – Advocating Reproductive Choices
Community engagement	– Forming women's groups: UHI, Pahel – Orientation of community members: Karuna Trust – Community-based monitoring: PFI – Community mobilization: Parivartan, Project Concern International – Community mobilization and monitoring: PSS
Focus on generating demand for specific elements of QoC	– Improving continuum of care: Integrated Family Health Initiative – Constellation of services: systematic screening: Population Council pilot
External monitoring to enhance accountability of the programme for QoC	– Quality assessment studies (medical audits): Ujjwal Project – External monitoring of private clinics by FOGSI: Ujjwal Project – Monitoring of sterilization camps: HealthWatch – Role of media: research – Social audit of failures and complications: research
Internal monitoring	– Data for monitoring: UHI – QACs established by Supreme Court guidance
Harnessing the private sector to increase clients' choice of providers	– Social franchising: PSI, HLFPPT, Janani/DKT – Private sector for postpartum IUCD: UHI – Social marketing: PSI, HLFPPT
Research on consequences of poor QoC to support advocacy	– Incidence of poor health outcomes – Poor RH of contraceptive users – Discontinuation of contraceptive use – High unmet need and its impact on health

9.3 Clients at the Centre of Quality of Care

9.3.1 Client Perspectives

Respect and dignity: Women should be treated with dignity and respect, which includes women's access to every possible method of FP, good counselling services, and efficient follow-up care. To make this possible, there is a need to define a framework of dignity in the context of QoC. At the same time, it is important to understand the outcomes of lack of dignity. What does lack of dignity mean for accessing contraceptive method choice? Exploratory research may be needed to understand this better.

Measuring quality: There is a need to create guidelines for measuring QoC by disrupting the discourse on what measures we use for quality and how we measure it. There is a need to define a set of variables that measure quality from the client's perspective. Leaving aside the definition of quality, we must try to understand how women understand care, what it means to care, what women understand by dignity and quality, how they articulate it, how they define dignity, self-worth, etc. Within the QoC concept, what is the convergence or divergence among the concepts of "quality" and "care"? What do we call this construct and how do we define it?

Hard versus soft dimensions: Clinical definitions of quality are sharp and acute, often overlooking the softer dimensions. Quality of care is often equated with provision of services. We need to move beyond service provision to include the softer dimensions of QoC, including the health information needs of clients, the care process, etc. We need to make a distinction between clinical and non-clinical methods to understand QoC holistically. There is a need to review the focus on technical rather than just client issues for improving informed choice and quality in technical service provision.

Gender issues: We set the bar rather low when we think of QoC standards for services to women. One of the biggest challenges is gender disparity and norms. Women are not making health decisions for themselves or their families. In the absence of autonomy in decision making, they are accepting poor quality of services. Quality of care is a common concern when women and young people demand services (including SRH, abortion, and contraception).

User-generated data for measuring quality: We have tolerated poor QoC in many fields, including health care for women. We need to draw the circle little more narrowly. Perceptions of providers and communities are shaped by their experiences. Providers must understand and respect their clients' needs, attitudes, and concerns, and client perceptions are in turn affected by personal, social, and cultural factors. Thus, there is a need for developing user-generated quality standards for FP care. This can be achieved by conducting studies using a participatory research design and mixed methods (incorporating the views of service users into quality improvement initiatives) to develop a set of indicators that measure quality from clients' perspective.

9.3.2 Empowering Clients

Empowering clients involves enhancing women's autonomy and decision-making power as well as engaging men. Women are not a homogeneous group (some are unable to make decisions for themselves), and are often not able to make decisions regarding their health. Within the client-centred approach, there is a marketplace and women are making choices regarding FP and contraception. However, are women making their own health decisions or are these decisions being made for them by others? Where does the control lie and to what extent do women exercise that control? There is a need to study women's decision-making process and their decision-making power in FP use at the household level and identifying associated factors.

Currently, the responsibility of FP lies largely with women. This needs to change and men need to play an equal and more proactive role in decision making and adoption of FP. Family planning is for women as well as for men. Thus, engaging with men is important as they are also participants.

Some research projects in this regard might include:

1. Ethnographic research to understand women's decision-making power in FP use at the household level and identifying associated factors.
2. Exploratory research to define a framework of dignity in the context of QoC. What is the result of lack of dignity in seeking care? What does lack of dignity mean for choice in FP?
3. Participatory research to develop user-generated quality standards for FP care; understanding the convergence and divergence between "quality" and "care" in FP.

9.4 Empowering Young People to Demand Quality of Care

9.4.1 Service-Seeking Behaviour of Young People

The discourse on QoC needs to be broadened to include emergent needs of young people. Young women are the least empowered in seeking quality care, including seeking care for contraceptives. At the same time we need to understand what stops young men from seeking help for SRH issues. Often young people fear sharing information with service providers or seeking care for fear of being stereotyped or for fear of being shamed before their parents ("we'll tell your parents"). Deconstructing the stereotypes is important. Research questions in this regard include:

1. Evaluating the youth-friendliness of current health services through a study to investigate young people's experiences of using SRH services at clinics providing the Youth-Friendly Health Services (YFHS) programme.
2. Assessing the training and monitoring needs of service providers to address young people's needs for FP/contraception.

Young people also need counselling to make decision about their choices. However, it is not clear what kinds of information are transacted with young women and men; is this information able to shape their demand for quality? What are the training and monitoring needs of service providers to address young people's needs for FP/contraception?

9.4.2 Unpacking Youth-Friendly Health Services

There is a need to unpack the perceived barriers (embarrassment, feeling shy, fear of safety, fear of family finding out, and cost) to accessing FP services and demystifying them so that important elements of quality are placed within the YFHS programme. Is maintaining the privacy of clients part of providing quality care? There is a need for an evaluative study to investigate young people's experiences of using SRH services at clinics offering the YFHS programme.

9.5 Engaging Community

The community needs to be engaged both to influence societal norms and to mainstream its involvement towards enhancing demand for QoC (see Annexure 3).

9.5.1 Influencing Societal Norms

It is necessary to look into the values and nuances of service providers and our own value systems regarding quality and women's rights so that we provide the best care possible. Stigma is a common concern when women and young people demand SRH, abortion, and contraception services. This highlights the need for more work to be done on various socio-cultural aspects of improving quality.

There is a need to focus on communicating on important factors like age at marriage and pregnancy. What platforms work best for communicating these issues? it is important to systematically look at what is working and what is not. Adolescents in school spaces can be targeted for delaying age at marriage. There is a need to prepare women and men prior to important events (such as marriage or pregnancy) in their lives.

Providers at the lowest level need to be oriented towards QoC, as they are as disempowered as the clients they serve. Since providers and clients come from the same communities, training programmes for service providers and communities should focus on addressing gender norms and power gaps in the provision of QoC.

The discourse around quality should be broadly defined as the ethics of care. We need to focus on the ethics of care first, rather than just quality, as there is a need to disturb the power balance between providers and women clients and to recommend tactical ways in which we deal with quality. In nearly a decade, the *Indian Journal of Medical Ethics* has changed the discourse around ethics. Still, it is built around masculine perspectives. We need to build on women's perspectives in the context of the nuances of their lives so as to develop suitable measures of quality as we work on enhancing demand.

9.5.2 Mainstreaming Community Involvement

So far the research agenda has been centred on clinics, FP methods, and service provision. It needs to move towards mainstreaming community involvement to monitor quality and address people's needs for quality care. People's aspirations are socially determined to some extent, and the poorest communities these days have much more capacity to alter the conditions of their lives, which reflects the change in aspirations. There is a need to understand how much of a QoC lens we are using in current service and care provision. Consistent policy and advocacy efforts will help strengthen community accountability mechanisms.

The following research questions emerge in this regard:

1. What is the role of community mobilization in influencing social norms around age at marriage and conception?
2. How do we create collaborative spaces at the micro level between providers and the community?
3. How does community mobilization contribute to gender equality and improved acceptance and uptake of FP services? What are the various platforms available to enhance gender equity?

Dignity is an important component when women define quality. Therefore, there is a need to understand dignity in all its dimensions including what the lack of dignity is leading to. Community engagement is needed to change perceptions at scale. *Gram sabhas* (meeting of all adults who live in the area covered by the Panchayat) and panchayats (village council) provide community engagement spaces. However, it is not clear how much devolution of power is happening through these mechanisms. The community that cares and endeavours to provide better QoC must also not ignore the power of creating alliances with other gender rights movements.

Sometimes it is possible to create collaborative spaces at facilities, at the micro level between providers and community. One African experience shows that providers and the community together looked at the data available with them and identified issues that needed attention. For instance, analysis of hospital data on maternal deaths showed that more deaths were happening at night. Further investigations found that senior care providers were not present during night shifts. The problem was addressed by posting some senior providers in the night shift. This experience also led to development of the state accountability system.

9.6 Working with Other Sectors

There is a need to identify different platforms available for facilitating and strengthening community actions and assess whether they are sufficiently resourced. There may be possibilities for making alliances and creating spaces with other women's and gender movements to enhance gender equity. It may also be feasible to address violence against women issues through these movements. To allow for new voices, we need to work with new platforms of engagement. Alliances are important, with both formal and informal structures. Every alliance has its own agenda and mandate, so there is a need to find the points of intersectorality. We need to locate this conversation within other linked movements and domains of work and make QoC and gender equity everybody's issue by making them inclusive and constructive. Research questions that emerge in this respect include: How can alliances with other sectors help enhance gender equity? What are the available platforms and points of synergy?

Various ministries have introduced schemes and policies that have far-reaching benefits for people's health and well-being. There is a need to identify possible interconnections or linkages between the schemes of different ministries for larger and far-reaching outcomes and impact. For example, schools need to link seamlessly with government programmes focusing on health.

9.7 Communication for Enhancing Demand

There is a need to build a discourse on quality. Demand for FP itself does not exist fully; the demand for QoC is far from optimal. In the name of demand, sometimes we educate the client on what to expect. That does not fully convey the client's perspective; it is the educator's perspective. Therefore, there is a need to take forward the agenda based on the client's perspective. To enable women to create demand for good-quality services, we need to articulate what quality care looks like so that they can demand it. Several challenges need to be addressed: How do we create a language of QoC? What issues of language arise around what qualifies as quality? How do you give legitimacy to newly defined thoughts on quality? (see Annexure 4)

9.7 Communication for Enhancing Demand

Are there communication campaigns, or is there space for something big that helps shift norms from accepting poor quality to being intolerant about poor quality? For example, past campaigns like Balbir Pasha (built around a fictional character called Balbir Pasha, the campaign spread awareneed to HIV and AIDS by using a story board to place the character in various high-risk sexual situations, with unknown outcomes) (HIV/AIDS) and a current series titled "Main Kuch Bhi Kar Sakti Hoon" (an initiative that aims to challenge the prevailing social and cultural norms around family planning, early marriage, early and repeated pregnancies, contraceptive use among other issues) address the middle class. We can learn from campaigns that address violence against women to look at strategies and methods for bringing about normative change at scale. More research is needed to understand the quality of communication delivered to communities and clients. Measuring what is working and what is not (methods, approaches, messages) as well as becoming more strategic with our use of various media channels is required for planning future strategies. There is global evidence on the use of new media and social media for behaviour change. We need to look at available evidence, from India and internationally, to develop specific communication plans.

There is a need to develop and tailor messages for different audiences. We need to look at global evidence to see where respect and dignity are manifested in language and articulation. Media play an important role in shifting norms, discourse, and language. Several issues need consideration: How can the mass media support the creation of or enhance the demand for quality? How do we conduct a dialogue? Which medium is most effective and which audience should be targeted? Layering of communication within existing campaigns will help.

There is also a need to revisit/develop a communication strategy based on the theory of change for creating/enhancing demand over a longer period of time. We need to identify spaces, platforms, and existing public engagement opportunities which need broadening for communication on QoC. The following research questions might be taken up in this respect:

1. Explore cultural and linguistic expressions of QoC in FP.
2. Develop a theory of change for enhancing demand for QoC in FP.

9.8 Governance

There is now a need to move to the next level of QoC. This agenda should be owned by both state (government) and non-state actors (NGOs, donors, researchers, community-based organizations, media). Quality needs to become a governance issue. The government at the national level is accountable for providing services such as counselling, ensuring male involvement, providing products and services, and disseminating information. All care and services have to be provided within quality parameters defined by the government, the budgets for which must be provided. The Supreme Court judgments lay emphasis on "dignity". Although the court does not define "dignity", it focuses on aspects surrounding the concept.

Most policies are perfectly stated on paper; however, the implementation of those policies has serious gaps. For instance, witness the poor implementation of policies for increasing the age of marriage. There is a need to probe the underlying reasons for poor implementation. A comprehensive assessment of the powerful three-tier village/community-level governance system—self-help groups, panchayat raj institutions (local government institutions), and field-level workers—is also needed.

9.9 Accountability

Participants argued that several dimensions of accountability need attention—accountability for what and why, whose accountability, and to whom. In addition, there is a need to institutionalize programme accountability (Annexure 5).

9.9.1 Accountability for What and Why

The government, at national and state levels, is accountable for providing QoC and services. However, is the government clearly articulating its commitment to the rights of women, and is health, or more specifically FP and contraception, seen as a right? The health ministry is not willing to say that health is a right. However, in Karnataka, health as a right is well articulated and promoted on billboards and other communication materials. So there is cause for optimism.

Since the government is a signatory to many global treaties that promote client rights as well as dignity, concentrated efforts can be made to track adherence to and progress against commitments made at the national and international levels.

The Supreme Court in its latest order has asked for quarterly reports from the MoHFW, and several aspects of QoC are covered in that order. We need to understand how it will work. Based on the Supreme Court judgment, what aspects of quality are DQACs being asked to report on? There is a need to plug in monitoring data. We must use the Supreme Court judgment to revive the DQAC.

Going forward, we should also be mindful that government is committed to recruiting 48 million new users of contraception during the period 2012–2020, which also demands providing QoC for achieving impact.

9.9.2 Whose Accountability and to Whom

Are the current approaches and measures of quality sufficient to ensure provider accountability to clients for good-quality services? Caregiving is a reciprocal process. Quality of care is not just about what is happening to women and clients who seek services, but also about (women) providers who provide care and services.

9.9 Accountability

The NHM has included community monitoring as one of the pillars of accountability. The government is experimenting with community monitoring. However, we have not done a good job of analysing the available data and putting it before government. Also, case studies on our experiences with community monitoring would help understand the process and stakeholders. Jan Samwad is also a forum where communities and providers can understand each other's issues.

There is also an opportunity for pilot programmes on the role of community-based monitoring in enhancing accountability for quality. For instance, Advance Family Planning has piloted district working groups with the district collector as the chair. Other departments are also involved. We need to see what the experience was. The role of community self-help groups is important as women are not sufficiently empowered. We also need to understand what our level of preparedness as accountability groups is. What kind of community institutions do we require to strengthen accountability as community members experience unequal power relations? In addition, tools and indicators needs to be simple, transparent, and easy to understand so that people are able to use them for measuring quality and facilitate community action.

There is a need for community-based research. The space for community has been gradually diminishing. There is a need to protect that space. The community needs to be directly involved in the process of change. The community is not represented in QACs. The role of community-based mechanisms like the VHNSCs or RKSs is also not clear in this regard. Community monitors are placed on an unequal level compared to providers. They also do not have technical knowledge with regard to clinical methods. Tools need to be simple and transparent.

Some RKSs meet regularly and others do not meet. Is the RKS functioning, and what is the impact? What are the barriers? Why have they failed? There is a need for advocacy for greater effectiveness of VHNSCs and RKSs, and also for greater space for community institutions such as panchayats and gram sabhas. Where do these bodies work effectively and where do they not work, and why? What is their output? What would be needed to sustain them? There are a lot of scattered experiences, nationally and internationally. There is a need to synthesize these experiences. Having foregrounded the issues, we need to assess whether they have resulted in change.

Besides government programmes, private sector accountability for QoC also needs to be strengthened. The private sector provides 80% of the health services and a significant proportion of non-clinical FP services. What is the responsibility of the government as a steward? So far, perceptions of clients and communities on QoC have been provided by the private sector. Going forward, the private sector will be a major player in FP. There is a need to focus on the supply side as well.

9.9.3 Institutionalizing Accountability

There is a need to strengthen accountability systems. Internal monitoring often does not work, and therefore the possibility of external monitoring needs to be explored. Independent bodies at the national level monitor quality; for example, the report of the Comptroller and Auditor General was shared with state governments. The audit results revealed that the institutional framework for implementation of quality assurance programme was either not in place or was not effective. The Report also noted low number of internal and external assessments of health facilities, inadequate reporting, and non-evaluation of key performance indicators. However, no action was taken on it. Should there be an independent body such as the Comptroller and Auditor General for monitoring? The Niti Aayog is also trying to enhance accountability. Further, civil society organizations and NGOs could be trained to negotiate. We also need to identify the characteristics of a successful QA system. What is the experience globally? What has worked? What would it cost? How scalable is it? For example, Indonesia has implemented a pilot and is trying to expand it to all its districts. This programme may provide clues on how QA should be looked at.

The following research questions emerge:

1. Scattered experiences, national and international, need to be synthesized. Having identified the issues, we need to assess whether they have resulted in change.
2. In which contexts do institutional mechanisms work and where do they not work, and why? What is their output? What would be needed to sustain them?

Monitoring and evaluation systems, in addition to capturing the data, also need to tell the story behind those numbers. Often data is presented to share the government's targets in service delivery, and do not focus on the quality of services. A comprehensive dashboard of indicators is required for people to know the range of FP choices available to them.

9.10 Advocacy

Applying pressure on the health system can affect the behaviours of service providers and caregivers simultaneously by changing the systems that guide their work to achieve quality care. Therefore, advocacy for QoC is essential (see Annexure 6).

A broader understanding of the context for QoC is needed. It is important to understand where QoC advocacy fits in the larger FP advocacy agenda. What role does it play in changing the quality landscape in FP? When it comes to QoC, a sense of urgency of tasks is missing. There are lessons from various parts of the country which need to be studied to understand the situation and the reasons for the lack of priority accorded to QoC. We do not know the intricacies of decision making. What is the process of decision making and what barriers does it face? Research must lead to some advocacy. Is there an opportunity for the research community to act as influencers? What are the possible platforms and opportunities?

9.10.1 Evidence Base for Advocacy

The concept and practice of evidence-based policy making insists that properly developed public policy draws on the best available evidence. We do not have enough evidence from national surveys such as NFHS and the National Sample Survey. There is a need to build institutional capacity to study, monitor, and evaluate QoC.

There is sufficient evidence of good QoC practices. However, we are missing evaluation data on many aspects which can be used for advocacy in support of the demand for QoC: (*a*) community-based delivery of contraceptives by ASHAs; (*b*) QoC for IUDs delivered at various levels of the health system—SCs (sub centre), PHCs, CHCs, and district hospitals—and the reasons for discontinuation; (*c*) QoC delivered in the private sector; data on social marketing and the framework for QoC; (*d*) epidemiological data on contraception-induced morbidities and discontinuation rates; (*e*) data on facility readiness; (*f*) analysis of DQAC reports; (*g*) quality of counselling; and (*h*) QA of commodities.

What is considered valid data in QoC? Where is the centre of data generation and who is generating this data? Can studies based on user-generated data and qualitative narratives be considered valid? The auditing of health services from a user perspective would generate useful information on QoC and people's experiences with care. There is a need to empower users to generate their own data (user-controlled, user-gathered data on QoC). What more data or information is needed to build upon existing studies that is currenlty not being captured? For example, women are not a homogeneous group; not all belong to the same category and their needs and decision-making ability also vary. Their diverse experiences can be used for advocacy. There is a gap between what is getting measured and what policy formulators are focusing on.

Evidence needs to be built around clients' own conceptualization of care and their idea of risk. The challenge is—how do we make this relevant to them? Do we have the right tools for this purpose, as well as for client satisfaction surveys? How do we understand women's experience in the context of care and provider empathy? The National Sample Survey Organization provides information on the use of the services of private providers. This data needs to be unpacked. We need ethnographic research on clients' choices, on why women choose a particular method or specific suppliers, the influence of community forces, family influence, personal preferences, and contraceptive morbidities and side effects. How do these choices differ between educated and uneducated women? Is the provider making decisions on their behalf?

9.10.2 Process of Advocacy

There is a need to advocate for QoC as a human right, as stated in Indian jurisprudence, i.e., in the context of concepts such as enforceability, violence etc.. A cross-legal analysis: PNDCT (Pre-Conception and Pre-Natal Diagnostic Techniques (PCPNDT) Act, 1994), VAW (Protection of Women from Domestic Violence Act 2005) etc. can be done to see how quality is articulated or stated in these guidelines and documents. A possible research area is on designing advocacy strategy: we need a theory of change for advocacy in support of demand for QoC in FP. What is the outcome we are looking for? What are the intermediary measures? How is the system learning from adverse events following family planning procedures?

How do we use advocacy with the recent Supreme Court judgment on QoC? How do we scale it? How do we make it a governance issue? There are several elements within the QoC framework proposed by the Supreme Court judgment which the government needs to take into account. The Supreme Court judgment can be used for creating a disruptive discussion around QoC and bringing forth issues that do not show up at this point.

Building the momentum for advocacy on QoC issues requires broader conversations. Can we join other players (those engaged in activism around violence, agency, and empowerment)? If these voices come together, the impact may be higher. However, each of these groups has a different set of normative issues; for instance, FP addresses changing social norms, gender equity, and so on. We can learn from other advocacy efforts such as that addressing gender-based violence, where research has been used effectively. We may wish to build alliances with the gender movement.

9.11 Service Provision

The consultation focused on enhancing demand for QoC. However, the participants repeatedly made references to the need for attention to service provision. The following comments were made.

9.11.1 Health System

Underlying universal access to QoC is respect for women's rights, human rights, and the right to health. We need to look at QoC for other health programmes also, such as tuberculosis. Selective improvements in FP cannot be made without strengthening health system. There is need to implement the IPHS. It is necessary to work at both state and district levels. To what extent is the health system geared towards addressing women's health needs? The universal health coverage approach is a good opportunity to address women's right to health. Under a decentralized approach to universal health coverage, actions may be taken at both the national and subnational levels. Women's right to health can be incorporated in the universal health coverage approach through advocacy and capacity building.

Additional evidence is needed on health workers' understanding of gender, as the power imbalance between service providers and women clients affects the quality of service provision. It is important to build their understanding on gender issues to help them better address the complexity of clients' care-seeking behaviour and decision-making context. For example, we need to understand why health service providers are not discussing side effects with clients.

Where does QoC fit in? How do we try to move this discussion from issues of access and provision of services to improvement of QoC? Quality of services is important for enhancing the demand for FP. Quality is often equated with provision; however, achieving a certain level of facility (infrastructure, supplies and services) is needed to provide QoC and induce demand for services. What can be done in the absence of public health systems?

Health system support systems are important. Supply forecasting mechanisms will help maintain a supply chain of products and services. Quality delivered may not be quality received. Therefore, there is a need to improve training methodology to enhance the skills of service providers in client interactions. In addition, there is a need to develop a career trajectory for the workforce to keep them motivated to provide quality care and services.

Time is an important factor in determining how much attention a client gets at the service delivery point and how much time a provider is able to assign to each client. Given the volume of clients, time emerges as a challenge. There is a need for a realistic assessment of what the provider can offer and what the client is willing to invest in terms of time. Thus, it is important to determine what needs to happen at points of transaction between the provider and the client. More needs to happen before a client reaches a service delivery point to seek care. It is necessary to look at traditional media and mass media approaches and a whole range of other approaches. The government keeps highlighting its provision of free services. How does that affect QoC?

Different programmes are offered at different points, but we need to follow one gold standard in FP QoC for women and young people. What is this gold standard? How do we agree on a common set of parameters?

The use of financial incentives to promote FP and method choice is another important area of research. Is this approach distorting the method choice? Or is it increasing the acceptance of other methods? How do incentives disturb expenditure and budget patterns? And how do provider incentives influence provider behaviour —these are important questions for research.

9.11.2 Empowering Providers

Provider perspectives and perceptions are important topics of study in improving the QoC experience for clients. As discussed in an earlier section, the act of seeking a service is an indicator of client empowerment. Therefore, the point of contact (health facility, provider) should also be empowering to reinforce people's faith in the system. Empathy at providers' end is critical. The service provider needs to be made part of research processes. Acknowledging the high degree of pressure on women providers, there is a need to understand the challenges and gaps at their end. Is it the prerogative of an ASHA alone to change the paradigm of service seeking? Client interaction flow and popular gold standards of quality need to be redefined. There is a need to shift norms within the provision of services and to relook at the gold standards of service. This may involve helping service providers to unlearn the old and develop a new definition of quality care. How do we instil a sense of pride in all service delivery? How is it that certain people/sectors are able to do this successfully? There is a need to learn from other sectors and institutions. The right to health needs to be integrated into the perspective of demanding QoC. Provider focus in enhancing demand is important. Some providers perceive that people need their services; therefore, they get what is provided by the service provider. This mindset needs to be changed by educating providers and encouraging them to think in terms of clients' perspectives. The principal research question in this area is therefore: What are the factors that affect providers' motivation, perceptions, expectations, and relationships with clients?

9.12 Conclusion

Issues affecting QoC extend beyond the service provider setting, influencing clients before they arrive to seek services. Important determinants that affect demand for QoC include the client's agency and autonomy, gender norms, socio-cultural factors, the costs of seeking quality care, myths and misconceptions about methods, and access to services. Clients' perspectives on the services they receive are an essential part of understanding and assessing QoC. These perspectives are shaped by cultural values and norms, past experiences, perceptions of the role of the health system, and interactions with service providers.

There are challenges that need to be addressed to create a supportive environment in which demand-side strategies can effectively improve access to quality FP services. It is, therefore, critical to identify emergent research, action, and advocacy priorities that would help enhance demand for quality, through which QoC in FP in India can be further improved and sustained.

References

Care India. (2013). Integrated family health intervention: Catalyzing change for healthy communities. CARE.

Essays, UK. (2013). Merrygold health network (HLFPPT) health and social care essay. Retrieved from http://www.ukessays.com/essays/healthandsocialcare/merrygoldhealthnetworkhlfpptheal thandsocialcareessay.php?cref=11

Futures Group. (2012). *IFPS technical assistance project, behaviour change communication activities and achievements—Lessons learned, best practices and promising approaches.* Gurgaon: Futures Group, ITAP.

Government of Odisha. (2013). *Impressions: The FP Odisha newsletter* 1 (no. 1). Directorate of Health and Family Welfare, Government of Odisha.

Karuna Trust. (2014). *Repositioning family planning at primary health centres. Quarterly Progress report*, Karuna Trust.

Marie Stopes International. (2014, 8 May). *Inquiry into the role of the private sector in promoting economic growth and reducing poverty in the Indo-Pacific region.*

Population Services International. (2014). *Pehel project report.*

Project Concern International. (2013). *Transforming lives: Sustaining the improvement of family health and sanitation in marginalized communities.* Parivartan: Bihar Community Mobilization Project, PCI Global.

Satia, J., & Chauhan, K. (2017). *Quality refresh: Taking stock and exploring new pathways to enhancing demand for quality of care in family planning in India.* Developing our research and advocacy agenda. Report of a national consultation, Jodhpur, January 16–17, 2017.

Satia, J., Chauhan, K., Bhattacharya, A., & Mishra, N. (2015). *Innovations in family planning: Case studies from India.* New Delhi: SAGE Publications.

Urban Health Initiative. (2014). *Annual report.*

Annexure 1
Delphi Questionnaire

Round 1

Research Agenda

QoC metrics: Although we have several frameworks for QoC, consensus about a parsimonious list of indicators perhaps has not emerged. How have studies and pilot programmes measured QoC and what can be learnt about use of some of these metrics at the macro level?

Client perceptions of quality: There is some evidence that there may be divergence between the ways studies perceive QoC and the ways women (and men) perceive QoC. Clearly, the interpersonal dimensions of QoC weigh heavily with clients, as they may not be able to assess the technical aspects of QoC. It would be useful to know: (*a*) what dimensions of QoC are important to clients; (*b*) what clients perceive as their benefits from receiving QoC; (*c*) how important is informed choice for them, and how does the social context determine the choice process; and (*d*) how to engage communities and women to ensure informed choice?

Myths and misconceptions: Some myths and misconceptions continue to persist, particularly regarding vasectomy. There is a need to look at why this is so and what can be done. Are there any successful experiences in this regard?

Respectful care: How can we ensure the dignity of women when they are availing of FP services? What is the current situation in this respect?

Factors enabling and motivating providers to provide QoC: Providers need a working environment that enables and motivates them to provide QoC. Although the FP programme in India has policies for a target-free approach, it is not clear how frontline staff—ANMs, PHCs—perceive this. What do providers think their benefit is in providing QoC? How has task shifting affected QoC? What factors affect providers' ability to provide QoC? How can these factors be strengthened?

Role of payments to acceptors of methods: As a considerable amount of the financial resources of the programme are devoted to payments (in lieu of wages foregone, etc.) to acceptors of sterilization and IUDs, there is a need to understand what role these payments play in the choice and acceptance process?

Client–provider interaction: What is the quality of client–provider interactions? How can it be improved?

Follow-up with clients: There is a need to improve follow-up with clients. When a woman seeks clinical services for FP and is found ineligible, then what options are offered? How well are complications managed?

Introducing additional methods: The government has recently decided to introduce the provision of DMPA in the public sector to expand the basket of contraceptive choices. What is the experience of DMPA introduction and what is the way forward?

Financial resources: There is evidence that measures to ensure QoC are underfunded. Some have argued that the money offered as incentives should instead be used to improve QoC. There is a need to develop better estimates of the funds needed to ensure the desired QoC and assess the extent of underfunding. While looking at current and needed financial resources for the FP programme, we also need to consider how well the existing financial allocations are utilized.

Monitoring QoC: Several recommendations have been made to monitor QoC, including the community monitoring system through NGOs, monitoring by VHNSCs and RKSs, use of mHealth for direct feedback from clients, and use of HMIS with a few indicators for quality. We need to look at various experiences of how QoC in FP is currently monitored through these mechanisms. It is not clear what the evidence is in this respect, and what more needs to be known. What kind of research would be needed?

Adolescent/youth: Adolescents and young people are currently underserved and have a high unmet need for spacing methods. The government has also begun to implement the RKSK initiative. What would be needed to ensure that adolescents/young people would be adequately served by high-quality contraceptive services?

Integrated RMNCH+A services: Family planning is an integral part of the RMNCH+A programme. However, often FP services are not adequately integrated with other services, particularly maternal and child health services. Would better integration improve QoC in FP services? If yes, how can we ensure such integration? What should be the constellation of services?

Quality of care to underserved and vulnerable populations in rural areas: Intervention research is required to develop cost-effective approaches to provide the desired level of QoC to underserved and vulnerable rural populations.

Quality of care for the urban poor: Intervention research is needed to find ways to reach the urban poor with high-quality care.

Quality of care to improve the continuation of spacing methods: There is some evidence that improving the QoC provided to current users of spacing methods will improve the continuation rate and reduce unmet need. Research is needed to develop effective ways to provide QoC to this group.

Factors determining QoC: What are the immediate factors contributing to QoC? What are the contributing factors affecting QoC? How to sustain QoC?

Market segmentation: How is the market segmented for different methods among the free, mixed-subsidized, and the private commercial sector? What are its implications?

Variation in QoC provided: Quality of care may vary considerably among different implementation models. It will be useful to determine the variance of different quality parameters in different FP service delivery models, like the public sector, NGO clinics, private sector accreditation sites, PPP sites, different parts of the private sector, etc.

Action Agenda

Activating QoC organizational mechanisms: The government has devised an organizational structure for QA comprising QA officers and QACs. Several states have taken action to institute this structure. What do we know about how they function and what can be done to activate them? How do we ensure that feedback from QA assessments is shared with district officials and, if necessary, with state officials?

Improving supply: Supplies are crucial for ensuring service quality. However, some studies have reported shortfalls in the availability of supplies. There is a need to continue to strengthen supply systems to ensure availability of contraceptives down to the village level. Odisha has tested a pilot commodities logistics management system which is now being scaled up.

Improving training: Training of both service providers and counsellors is critical to providing QoC. The government has taken action to strengthen specific competencies. There is a need to assess and improve competencies comprehensively. While looking at provider training, we should also consider medical and nursing education, as FP is neglected, particularly in private medical colleges.

Strengthening the role of ASHAs: The government has emphasized the role of ASHAs for community-level supply of pills, condoms, and ECPs. However, some studies have reported supply shortages, lack of motivation, and inadequate training as hampering these efforts. What do we know about remedial measures that work?

Enhancing accountability of the programme: Some have argued that the FP programme needs to become more accountable for the QoC it offers to clients and communities. The programme would need to assess QoC systematically and report the assessment results annually to all stakeholders.

Quality of care in the private sector: There is a need to improve the process of accreditation and the financing of private sector services to ensure the desired level of QoC in private sector services.

Periodic assessment of QoC: A system needs to be put in place to carry out periodic assessment of the QoC that is being provided to underserved and vulnerable populations. The NHSRC has begun the process of accreditation of private hospitals for the services they provide, including FP.

Advocacy Priorities

Commitment to QoC: There is a general perception that commitment to QoC among key stakeholders needs to be strengthened. Generally, pressure for quality comes from the "voice" and "choices" available to clients and communities. How can these forces be strengthened? Are there alternative ways to increase pressure for QoC, such as dipstick studies or a system to get feedback from clients?

Introducing additional methods: There has been some advocacy effort to introduce additional methods. To date the focus has been on DMPA. However, POP, LAM, and SDM may meet niche needs. Should advocacy efforts continue for their introduction?

Providing additional resources for FP: The government has pledged an additional USD2 billion for FP 2020. Should there be advocacy to provide more financial resources to improve access, availability, and QoC of FP?

Round 2
Research Agenda

Introducing additional methods: The government has recently decided to introduce the provision of DMPA in the public sector to expand the basket of contraceptive choices. What is the experience of DMPA introduction and what is the way forward?

Financial resources: There is evidence that measures to ensure QoC are underfunded. Some have argued that the money offered as incentives should instead be used to improve QoC. There is a need to develop better estimates of the funds needed to ensure the desired QoC and to assess the extent of underfunding. While looking at the current and needed financial resources for the FP programme, we need to also consider how well existing financial allocations are being utilized.

Monitoring QoC: Several recommendations have been made to monitor QoC, including the community monitoring system through NGOs, monitoring by VHNSCs and RKSs, use of mHealth for direct feedback from clients, and use of HMIS with a few indicators for quality. We need to look at various experiences as to how QoC in FP is currently monitored through these mechanisms. It is not clear what the evidence is in this respect and what more needs to be known. What kind of research would be needed?

Adolescent/youth: Adolescents and young people are currently underserved and have a high unmet need for spacing methods. The government has also begun to implement the RKSK programme. What would be needed to ensure that adolescents/young people are adequately served by high-quality contraceptive services?

Respectful care: How to ensure the dignity of women when they are availing of FP services? What is the current situation in this respect?

Client–provider interaction: What is the quality of client–provider interactions? How can it be improved?

Integrated RMNCH+A services: Family planning is an integral part of the RMNCH+A programme. However, often FP services are not adequately integrated with other services, particularly maternal and child health services. Will better integration improve QoC in FP services? If yes, how to ensure such integration? What should be the constellation of services?

Monitor QoC in FP service delivery sessions.

Annexure 2
Clients at the Centre of Quality of Care

An understanding of QoC is practically non-existent among the end users of FP services. Most clients are not aware of the components of QoC, their own rights, choices, etc. Several studies show that the status of QoC is poor. Cases also continue to be reported in the media. Various aspects of QoC need to be considered:

Respectful care: It is important to understand what clients perceive as necessary to ensure the dignity of women when they are availing of FP services. To assess the importance of this element, an understanding of the current situation in this regard as well as the importance attached to this aspect by women is needed.

Client–provider interaction: The quality of client–provider interactions often determines client satisfaction. There is growing belief that client–provider joint decision making improves QoC. However, even without this, the service provided may be excellent and safe, particularly in the case of clinical services.

Informed choice: It is not clear how important informed choice is for clients, or how the social context determines the choice process. It is necessary to understand these aspects to describe the process by which empowered individuals arrive at informed decisions on whether to obtain or decline contraceptive service, what contraception to select, and whether to seek and follow up on a referral, or to further consider the matter.

Technical dimensions of QoC: With regard to client perceptions of quality, interpersonal dimensions weigh heavily as compared to technical dimensions. Studies have shown that substandard services may be perceived as good-quality services particularly by poor and underserved clients. Often there is a wide difference between client perception and the actual levels of technical quality of services provided in public health facilities.

Influence of agency and community norms: It is important to understand how community norms and values affect client perceptions on the above aspects. How does the agency and autonomy of women affect their perceptions of QoC, particularly with regard to informed choice? What can be done to influence social context?

Rating of services: To improve QoC, it would be useful if clients were able to rate and comment on the services on a public forum not in the control of providers or policy makers. Clients could rate: (*a*) whether they received the FP service they came for; and (*b*) whether they would recommend the provider to a family member or neighbour or friend. There is a further need to investigate and derive a correlation between client assessment of quality and service delivery outcomes. Bringing to bear clients', especially women's, perspectives on what is important and what they expect from services will be critical. This will help in identifying the gaps and what needs to be done to meet clients' needs. It will make the process inclusive and bring in transparency and accountability.

Enhancing demand for QoC in adolescent/youth FP services: Adolescents and young people are currently underserved and have a high unmet need for spacing methods. This group has different priorities which need to be understood and addressed. The needs of married and unmarried people are different. Married young couples, although covered under the programme, need education and friendly services should they wish to delay the first pregnancy or space successive pregnancies. The unmarried sexually active population has the highest unmet need, defined as: (*a*) sexually active; (*b*) wanting to prevent pregnancy; and (*c*) not using an FP method. They need non-judgemental, confidential services. The unmarried group of clients is mostly neglected. Therefore, separate studies of married and unmarried clients would be needed.

Annexure 3
Community Engagement for Demanding Quality of Care in Family Planning

Active involvement of affected populations has been recognized as one of the key principles in improving QoC and ensuring human rights in the provision of FP/contraceptive services. Several efforts have focused on engaging with communities for increasing contraceptive prevalence. For instance, the media has been used to promote understanding of the benefits of FP by either limiting family size or spacing births, with a view to increasing the coverage of FP. However, the focus on enhancing demand for QoC has been very limited.

Empowering communities to demand QoC can make a difference. For instance, a programme of community education and use of mass media in Indonesia was positively associated with clients' preparation of questions and questioning behaviour during FP consultations, indicating that a combined community education and mass media approach can improve client communication with providers and improve the quality of FP counselling.

A scoping review of participatory approaches involving community and health care providers in FP/contraceptive information and service provision showed that community participation continues to be inadequately addressed in large-scale programmes. The review identified three types of approaches: (*a*) establishment of new groups such as health committees; (*b*) collaboration with existing community structures; and (*c*) operationalization of tools to facilitate collaboration among the community and health care providers for QI. There is insufficient research to develop mechanisms of community participation in different contexts for demanding QoC in FP.

Some have argued that community participation is seen as a means to an end for programmes to meet their objectives. The goal of community engagement could also be seen as one where community members serve as champions and advocates for sustained community programmes.

There may be a need to strengthen the capacity of ASHAs to address information asymmetry between clients/community members and service providers in enhancing demand for QoC in FP. Finally, there is a need to create greater awareness of clients' rights and QoC among all stakeholders. The key message is that the failure to honour clients' rights would mean that clients would experience substandard quality that would lead to contraceptive discontinuation, unintended pregnancies, avoidable morbidity, and even mortality.

Gender relations and norms within the community determine women's ability to practise contraception or demand QoC. The rights and empowerment aspects of quality for women are completely undermined. Involving men and engaging them as partners to ensure an enabling environment at the community level will encourage the development of effective partnerships between men and women. Interventions to influence gender relations in the context of FP include male engagement involving gender counselling and focus on spacing methods of contraception. For instance, male engagement was sought through a multi-session intervention delivered to men but inclusive of their wives. Many NGOs have used male workers to promote the engagement of men either in practising contraception themselves or in enabling and supporting their wives to use contraception. Community-based initiatives can be effective in mobilizing communities, empowering women, and promoting community dialogue and change on issues of gender equality (e.g., the PRACHAR Project).

The goal of this session was to propose research issues/topics to effectively engage communities for renewed emphasis on enhancing demand for QoC in FP, and to enhance the quality of FP services for reducing unmet need and ensuring human rights.

Interventions/Research for Enhancing Community Engagement to Demand Quality of Care

Our review of research and interventions to improve community engagement reveals that the following programmes focused on enhancing demand for QoC through community engagement:

Community engagement:

- Forming/strengthening women's groups: UHI, Pahel
- Orientation of community members: Karuna Trust
- Community-based monitoring: PFI
- Community mobilization and monitoring: PSS, Population Council.

Enhancing gender equity:

- Education of couples and expansion of the role of husbands: CHARM
- Advocating Reproductive Choices.

Emergent Research Priorities and Questions

- What are the community perceptions about the QoC currently being delivered and what changes would they like to see?
- Can community dialogues help to shift social norms and enable QoC in FP? What other mechanisms including using information and communication technology can be utilized? How do these shifts at the community level influence communication, decision making, and FP use at the couple or household level?
- How does the social context determine the choice process? How can we engage communities and women to ensure informed choice?
- How can the community help to monitor the work of QACs in priority states to provide planning, implementation, and monitoring support to the FP programme?
- What are the most effective social mobilization strategies to increase the age of marriage and raise awareness on delaying the first birth?
- What effective mechanisms exist for influencing gender relations in the context of FP? How can information and communication technology be harnessed for this purpose? Can they be scaled up in a cost-effective manner?
- What effective mechanisms exist to expand service delivery of FP products and services through innovative partnerships with the private sector and civil society?

Annexure 4
Interventions/Research for Creating Demand for Quality of Care by Clients

Our review of research and interventions revealed that the following programmes focused on enhancing demand for QoC by clients:

Client education and message reinforcement

- Helpline: Dimpa, Saadhan (PSI)
- Complementary helpline service with FAQs: Pahel, PSI
- Use of mHealth platform to assist clients for informed choice
- Comprehensive campaign: IFPS
- QoC as a part of FP demand generation communication.

Client feedback

- Empowering clients to demand QoC using mobile technology: C3
- Improving management: including patient feedback: Karuna Trust
- Follow-up mechanism for client feedback: Ipas
- Client satisfaction surveys: Ujjwal Project.

Focus on generating demand for specific elements of QoC

- Improving continuum of care: Integrated Family Health Intervention (IFHI)
- Constellation of services: Population Council pilot on systematic screening.

Emergent Research Issues/Questions

The client-centred approach is yet to take root in government and private FP programmes. So this area may require the utmost priority. Information asymmetry between clients and service providers creates problems in demanding QoC. Rising socio-economic status of clients, particularly women, as well as information technology and communication media advances including social media, offer opportunities to reduce information asymmetry.

Quality of care perceptions: What dimensions of QoC are important to clients? Clearly, interpersonal dimensions of QoC will weigh heavily with clients as they may not be able to assess the technical aspects of QoC. It would be useful to know: (*a*) what dimensions of QoC are important to clients; (*b*) what the current situation is with respect to upholding the dignity of women when they are availing of FP services; (*c*) how good is the follow-up with clients, and how well complications are managed; (*d*) what options are provided when a woman seeks clinical services for FP and is found ineligible; (*e*) how important informed choice is for clients; (*f*) what clients perceive as their benefits from receiving QoC. In this study, questions should be asked to men also to explore how clients (both men and women) perceive QoC in the context of rights.

Intervention research: What will be needed to empower clients to demand QoC? As it is not clear what works in this respect, there is a need to develop and test alternative ways as well as evaluating their impact on the demand for QoC.

Adolescent/young people: What would be needed to ensure that adolescents/young people can demand high-quality contraceptive services?

- *Implementation*: The government has an adolescent and youth policy as well as a service delivery strategy. The government has also begun to implement the RKSK initiative. The study should identify the problems/constraints in these programmes from the clients' perspectives.
- *Organizing service delivery*: The SRH needs of adolescents/youth can be ascertained from studies, but their preferences for access need to be studied. Also, information is needed from providers about social contexts and biases that pose challenges (and maybe some facilitating factors). Further, there is a need to understand the barriers to provision of quality services from the perspective of this group and how these barriers can be addressed.
- *Commercial channels*: Social marketing/commercial markets are growing for ECPs/condoms and pills. There is a need to study how adolescents/youth access these channels, as there are no separate protocols for FP for adolescents. Recent policy on including contraceptives under price control would also improve use.

Annexure 5
Enhancing Programme Accountability for Quality of Care

Some have argued that creating demand may have only suboptimal results unless this demand is translated into pressure on service providers to respond through enhanced accountability of programmes for QoC. It is felt that at present, the accountability of the FP programme is defined very vaguely, mostly limited to numbers, i.e., achieving the target; none exists for QoC. Broadly, demand for QoC can be transmitted to the service delivery system though increased voice for clients and communities, and choice of providers/option to exit for clients.

We can strengthen horizontal accountability through internal monitoring, including QACs and parliamentary hearings. It is often argued that it would be more efficient if citizens and their associations directly held duty bearers responsible for their acts or liable to face sanctions. Among other measures, this includes civil suits or criminal charges for violations of national guidelines, shadow reports, and investigative news reports. Finally, accountability can be enhanced through alliances between citizens and public institutions to improve the oversight of state and institutional actions such as participatory budgeting, civil society representation on oversight committees, or community representatives on health committees.

The accountability framework under the NHM comprises a mix of community monitoring, external surveys, routine internal monitoring, and public reports. A limitation of these instruments is that currently they include very few indicators of QoC in FP.

External monitoring can strengthen the voice of clients and communities. Several recommendations have been made to monitor QoC including community monitoring systems through NGOs, monitoring by VHNSCs and RKSs, and use of mHealth for direct feedback from clients. Views on community monitoring vary. One view is that we should identify alternative ways to monitor quality, especially community-led monitoring. The NHM provides a framework for accountability of service providers through community participation that has been used in several states (for example, Maharashtra and Bihar). mHealth (IVRS) has also been used for community monitoring of health indicators, including QoC. One of the challenges cited in such studies is that it becomes difficult to segregate the FP experience from the broad array of health services monitored through community-based monitoring. Research is needed to generate evidence on results from these and many other innovative initiatives/pilots and the scalability potential thereof. Social audits, in some cases, have had limited impact even though findings are shared with stakeholders including programme managers and service providers. Legal accountability for QoC in sterilization services has enabled monitoring of QoC, but it does not suffice.

Some have felt that that community monitoring of the quality of clinical services is difficult. How would a community know if proper asepsis was maintained during surgery or if analgesia/sedation was adequate? The HMIS provides information on complications and failures of sterilization, and this system should work. Therefore, internal QA/monitoring/accountability/accreditation mechanisms need to be assessed and strengthened. It is not clear if a choice of providers or options to exit would improve QoC in public or private service delivery for FP. Data on the use of sources of services in national surveys indicates that clients seem to exercise their choice for different methods using a mix of public and private providers. However, the factors that have influenced these choices are not clear. The information and communication revolution as well as social media are providing opportunities to empower citizens and communities to demand accountability from public and private service providers or exercise their options of choice/exit.

Interventions/Research

Our review of the research and of interventions to improve QoC suggests that the following programmes focused on enhancing accountability for QoC in FP:
External monitoring to enhance accountability of the programme for QoC

– Monitoring of sterilization camps: HealthWatch
– Quality assessment studies (medical audits): Ujjwal Project
– External monitoring of private clinics by FOGSI: Ujjwal Project
– Role of media: research
– Social audit of failures and complications: research.

Internal monitoring

– Data for monitoring: UHI
– QACs established by Supreme Court guidance.

Harnessing the private sector to increase clients' choice of providers

– Social franchising: PSI, HLFPPT, Janani/DKT
– Private sector for PPIUCD: UHI
– Social marketing: PSI, HLFPPT.

Research Issues

Quality of Care metrics: We have several frameworks for QoC. However, a consensus about a parsimonious list of indicators has perhaps not emerged. It is important to build consensus on a set of indicators for QoC at all levels—from the district to the national level. It is also important to assess how the current set of indicators dilutes the focus on QoC. Also, we need to measure the reproductive rights element of FP (starting from achieving the desired family size, which is usually not covered in the frameworks).

Monitoring systems: There is a need to use a combination of approaches for monitoring of QoC, as one size does not fit all purposes. Many models, such as those listed here for external and internal accountability, have been tried in different states of the country. It would be useful to identify and document successful initiatives that have positively impacted end users and have the potential for scaling up. What are the methodologies and indicators of quality for FP and SRH services in these initiatives?

Accountability: Mostly, the FP programme does not contain formal mechanisms of accountability to the community. Hence the need to understand their effectiveness and impact on improving the quality of services provided to the clients. Internal audits, regular monitoring, and rapid surveys are already a part of the accountability framework under the NHM. This study should highlight what is required, where the gap is, what the constraints are, and how the system can handle proper accountability for both quantity and quality. Also, there is a need to specify how to report and at what forums and periodicity.

Annexure 6
Evidence-Based Advocacy to Support Demand for Quality of Care

There is a general perception that commitment to QoC among key stakeholders needs to be strengthened. The respondents of the Delphi study also identified strengthening commitment to QoC among key stakeholders as the major advocacy objective. Perhaps there is inadequate understanding of the consequences that clients face when they receive inadequate QoC, including those arising from unmet need for FP (unwanted or mistimed pregnancies and the consequences thereof). There is evidence that improved QoC increases facility utilization and reduces unmet need, and the adverse consequences of having too many, too close, and too early pregnancies are also widely known. However, the consequences of unwanted pregnancies (abortions, impact on maternal and child health) and mistimed pregnancies (suboptimal birth intervals, impact on maternal and child health) are underappreciated.

Successful advocacy requires that evidence for the criticality of the cause is advocated, along with an effective process of advocacy and mechanisms to implement the process.

Generally FP administrators prioritize increasing access over improving the quality of current services as long as these services are seen to be improving contraceptive prevalence. Some of these measures, such as adding new methods to the programme, also improve choice and prevalence. Increasing access is also justified as increasing equity. However, the trade-off between increasing access and improving quality shifts as near-universal access and high level of coverage are achieved. This point of inflection is not always clear unless either improving access does not improve coverage significantly, or improved coverage does not result in a corresponding improvement in prevalence. Therefore, evidence-based advocacy is necessary for increasing priority for improving QoC.

To support advocacy for prioritization of improving QoC, it is necessary that the benefits of improved QoC are comprehensively studied. Quality of care not only reduces the side effects or complications arising out of contraceptive use, but also reduces their adverse impact on health. Clients experience an overall improved service experience and contraceptive use. The effects of poor QoC include the reverse of the above effects. Studies on the impact of improving QoC have focused on one or more of the above effects, but have not comprehensively studied them.

There is a need to understand whether the focus of advocacy efforts should be on enhancing demand for specific elements of QoC, or on the overall aspects. Further research is also needed to identify the most effective processes and methods as well as mechanisms for supporting effective advocacy for demand for QoC in FP by stakeholders.

Interventions/Research for Creating Demand for Quality of Care

Our review of research and interventions to improve QoC suggests that the following initiatives have focused on advocacy for QoC in FP. The initiatives mentioned below built the capacity of CSOs and FP advocates and catalysed their involvement, prepared and disseminated evidence-based advocacy materials, and enhanced collaboration between CSOs and government.

Advocating Reproductive Choices: Because of persistent weaknesses in the FP programme as well as reduced attention to FP, a group of health professionals and service delivery organizations came together to advocate for increased choices and strengthening the availability of contraception in India. The ARC, led by a secretariat, has ownership of this effort. It has built the capacity of stakeholders and has sought collaboration with the government, donors, and academic institutions in the form of technical support groups.

Population Foundation of India: The PFI has the long-standing mandate of advocating for FP and RH services. In 2011, PFI developed a strategic plan to reposition FP based on an analysis of the key drivers of population growth. It has focused most of its advocacy efforts on expanding choice and increasing resources for FP at the national level and in the states of Bihar and Uttar Pradesh—states with high unmet need.

- *Advance FP*: PFI works to increase contraceptive options and improve access to a wide range of contraceptive methods, with QoC at the centre. The work of JHPIEGO focuses on bringing about programmatic and policy-level changes to ensure access to quality in FP services. Pathfinder International advocates for the inclusion of FP into corporate social responsibility policies and increasing financial allocations year by year.
- *Advocacy for change*: PFI identified a range of "promising" strategies that would help reposition FP as a means of upholding the health and rights of women, men, and children. Under this effort, ASHAs, anganwadi workers, and panchayat raj institution members were sensitized through training to the need for repositioning FP, particularly birth spacing, in a block each in two districts of Bihar.

Annexure 6: Evidence-Based Advocacy to Support Demand ...

Repositioning FP: The Family Planning Association of India, with support from the IPPF, launched an advocacy initiative which mobilizes CSOs to reposition FP and to increase their dialogue with the government. The repositioning of FP implies a paradigm shift from an agenda that focuses on population stabilization to one where gender and rights, and a client-centred approach in the delivery of services, are given priority.

The efforts just mentioned are interrelated and strive towards the same goals. The mechanisms used in these approaches include forming a network of like-minded institutions by establishing a secretariat in one of the organizations. The network-led advocacy mechanisms comprise like-minded organizations that seek to pursue continued advocacy for a cause they believe in rather than making episodic efforts.

The methods of advocacy include the following:

- Developing advocacy tools including evidence building
- Synthesized evidence on effective interventions or "what works"
- Preparing brochures and other advocacy materials
- Advocacy with stakeholders, with donors, and dialogue and negotiation with key policy makers towards increasing budget allocation and expenditure for FP, increasing contraceptive choices, addressing policy barriers to improving the FP programme, and improving performance review mechanisms for FP in the state agenda
- Building the capacity of stakeholders to advocate for enhancing demand for QoC
- Awareness-building activities and cross-learning events.

Emergent Research Priorities and Questions

Impact: It would be useful to relate improvements in QoC to facility utilization, reduced quantum and severity of side effects or complications arising from contraceptive use, unmet need, reductions in unwanted and mistimed pregnancies and their adverse impact on maternal and child health, and overall client experience.

Perceptions of stakeholders on QoC: An in-depth study on this issue is important to find out the perceptions/views of programme managers and clients/communities regarding the benefits of improved QoC as well as the consequences of poor QoC.

Increasing commitment to QoC: Who are the key stakeholders who can influence the programme to provide QoC (people's representatives, interest groups, professional associations, district administrators, private service providers, others)? What are the different ways to increase pressure for QoC, such as dipstick studies, or a system to get feedback from clients with key stakeholders.

Advocacy process: Do advocacy efforts that focus on specific constituents of QoC work better as compared to focusing on the overall aspect (or combining various elements)? What are the advantages?

Motivating service providers: How effective would it be to create champions or offering recognition/accreditation to motivate providers to improve QoC? Is there a value to directly influencing service providers by using communication technologies including social media?